D1127104

Oral Cancer:

The Dentist's Role in Diagnosis, Management, Rehabilitation, and Prevention

Dedication

To my parents, who gave me so much and asked so little.

R. A. Ord

I dedicate this book to my mother and father. Their limitless support, understanding and encouragement have allowed me to pursue my goals throughout my life. I also hope that those who contributed to my professional development and education see in this book some return on the debt I owe to them for their efforts.

R. H. Blanchaert

Oral Cancer:
The Dentist's Role in Diagnosis, Management, Rehabilitation, and Prevention

Edited by:

Robert A. Ord, DDS, MD, MS
Professor
Department of Oral and Maxillofacial Surgery
Baltimore College of Dental Surgery
Dental School
University of Maryland at Baltimore

Greenebaum Cancer Center
University of Maryland Medical Center
Baltimore, Maryland

and

Remy H. Blanchaert, Jr, MD, DDS
Assistant Professor
Department of Oral and Maxillofacial Surgery
Baltimore College of Dental Surgery
Dental School
University of Maryland at Baltimore

Greenebaum Cancer Center
University of Maryland Medical Center
Baltimore, Maryland

Quintessence Publishing Co, Inc
Chicago, Berlin, London, Tokyo, Paris, Barcelona,
São Paulo, Moscow, Prague, and Warsaw

Library of Congress Cataloging-in-Publication Data

Oral cancer: the dentist's role in diagnosis, management, rehabilitation, and prevention /
edited by Robert A. Ord and Remy H. Blanchaert, Jr.
      p. ; cm
  Includes bibliographical references and index.
  ISBN 0-86715-357-1
  1. Mouth—Cancer. 2. Dentistry. I. Ord, Robert A. II. Blanchaert, Remy H.
  [DNLM: 1. Mouth Neoplasms—diagnosis. 2. Dentist's Practice Patterns. 3. Mouth
Neoplasms—therapy. WU 280 O643 1999]
  RC280.M6 O727 1999
  616.99'431—dc21   99-040839

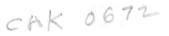

quintessence
books

© 2000 Quintessence Publishing Co, Inc

Quintessence Publishing Co, Inc
551 Kimberly Drive
Carol Stream, Illinois 60188

Printed in China

Contents

Foreword

The complexity of today's scientific and professional world, and the nature of health problems yet to be solved or adequately addressed in industrialized countries of the developed world, are such that individual expertise does not suffice. Rather, an array of talents, knowledge, backgrounds, and skills are required. In many cases this is true not only for the advancement of relevant knowledge, but also for the application of existing knowledge in the health care setting. In their preface the editors point out the necessity for a team approach to oral cancer. The relatively small size of dental schools as research and health care enterprises, and the diversity inherent in their educational tasks, dictate that only a limited number of unresolved oral and craniofacial health issues can be addressed by group effort in any one institution. The University of Maryland's Dental School is fortunate to have faculty and colleagues working together on our campus to address the problems of oral cancer, all the way from the laboratory bench to an effect in the community. This book is the product of that team approach.

In preparation for its efforts in the last decade of the twentieth century, the US Institute of Dental and Craniofacial Research (then NIDR) titled its long-range plan "Broadening the Scope," in recognition of the great needs posed by conditions, like oral cancer, which affect the oral and craniofacial region but which had not traditionally been the major concerns of dental research and practice. Despite the great progress that had been made in achieving improved oral health for US citizens by professional attention to conventional dental concerns, such as caries and periodon-tal diseases, mortality and morbidity from oral cancer had not been similarly alleviated. Now, at the beginning of the twenty-first century, this is still the case. In fact, it appears to be getting worse, perhaps at least in part due to improvements in diagnosis and tracking.

Because they are so well positioned to be effective, it is critical that oral health professionals take up the challenge of understanding, preventing, diagnosing, and treating oral cancer as regular and important features of their practices. This book will be of great value to those professionals who will get more involved. It covers everything from where the diseases are, what they are, and how they are diagnosed and treated, to important strategies for prevention and the impact on both individuals and society. It does so in an easy-to-read introductory format, but it also provides enough real meat and plenty of references to satisfy more sophisticated needs.

I am immensely pleased and proud that our faculty are providing this service to all oral health care professionals and, therefore, to those they serve. But I also am especially happy that this team has come together at this place and time, when incidence of oral cancer in Maryland is higher than the US average and its mortality rate is among the highest of all the states. I gratefully expect the authors of this text to have significant impact on the problem here.

Richard R. Ranney, DDS, MS
Dean
Baltimore College of Dental Surgery
Dental School
University of Maryland at Baltimore

Preface

With approximately 30,000 new cases of oral and oral pharyngeal cancer diagnosed each year in the United States, oral cancer is an important public health issue. This type of cancer is unique in that the dental profession can play a major role in its management. It is estimated that between 65% and 75% of patients with oral cancer will initially present to a dentist. Dentists are involved in the diagnosis, treatment, rehabilitation, reconstruction, and prevention of oral cancer. In addition, dental specialists are actively researching the molecular biology of oral cancer, while public health dentists are lobbying for more government-funded tobacco control and other preventive programs.

This book is written specifically for the dental health care provider, including dental students, general dentists, dental specialists, and hygienists; it focuses on the major contributions that the dental profession can make in the field of oral cancer health care delivery. While the general dental practitioner may see only one or two patients with oral cancer in a practice lifetime, the devastating consequences of a missed or delayed diagnosis mandate that all dentists become expert in the diagnosis of such cases. Through its role in the functional rehabilitation of oral cancer patients, the dental profession also contributes significantly to the quality of life of this patient population. Interventions such as tobacco cessation counseling are yet another means by which dental health care providers can effect a positive change in the health status of an entire community. There is truly no other disease in which the dental profession can have such a vital impact.

Experience has shown that the optimal management of oral cancer requires a "team" of interested and dedicated providers. This book was written by the members of such a team at the University of Maryland at Baltimore. It is the editors' hope that all dentists who read this book will regard themselves as an integral part of a team working toward the universal goal of the optimization of health care delivery to the oral cancer patient.

We wish to express deep and sincere thanks to the contributing authors, whose devotion to oral cancer care—something we witness daily—is evident in the quality of their chapters. Special thanks also goes to Ms Zina McKee for her good humor and diligence in assisting the work of the editors. A final thank you goes to Quintessence Publishing for the advice and help they provided in the preparation of this book.

Robert A. Ord, MD, DDS, MS
Remy H. Blanchaert, Jr, MD, DDS

Contributors

Marvin Baer, DDS, MS
Associate Professor
Department of Restorative Dentistry
Dental School
University of Maryland at Baltimore
Baltimore, Maryland

Remy H. Blanchaert, Jr, MD, DDS
Assistant Professor
Department of Oral and Maxillofacial
  Surgery
Baltimore College of Dental Surgery
Dental School
University of Maryland at Baltimore

Greenebaum Cancer Center
University of Maryland Medical Center
Baltimore, Maryland

Barbara A. Conley, MD
Senior Investigator
Cancer Therapy Evaluation Program
National Cancer Institute
National Institutes of Health
Bethesda, Maryland

Ricardo Della Coletta, DDS, PhD
Assistant Professor
Department of Oral Pathology
University of Campinas, Piracicaba
São Paulo, Brazil

Carl F. Driscoll, DMD
Assistant Professor
Department of Restorative Dentistry
Baltimore College of Dental Surgery
Dental School
University of Maryland at Baltimore
Baltimore, Maryland

M. Cara Erskine, MEd
Senior Speech Language Pathologist
Department of Rehabilitation Services
University of Maryland Medical Center
Baltimore, Maryland

Jacquelyn L. Fried, RDH, MS
Associate Professor
Department of Dental Hygiene
Dental School
University of Maryland at Baltimore
Baltimore, Maryland

Robert A. Ord, DDS, MD, MS
Professor
Department of Oral and Maxillofacial
  Surgery
Baltimore College of Dental Surgery
Dental School
University of Maryland at Baltimore

Greenebaum Cancer Center
University of Maryland Medical Center
Baltimore, Maryland

Mark A. Reynolds, DDS, PhD
Assistant Professor
Department of Oral and Maxillofacial
   Pathology
Baltimore College of Dental Surgery
Dental School
University of Maryland at Baltimore
Baltimore, Maryland

Miriam R. Robbins, DDS, MS
Division Head, Hospital Dentistry
Director, General Practice Residency
University of Maryland Medical Center

Assistant Professor
Department of Oral Health Care Delivery
Dental School
Baltimore College of Dental Surgery
University of Maryland at Baltimore
Baltimore, Maryland

John J. Sauk, DDS, MS
Professor and Chair
Department of Oral and Maxillofacial
   Pathology
Baltimore College of Dental Surgery
Dental School
University of Maryland at Baltimore

Greenebaum Cancer Center
University of Maryland Medical Center
Baltimore, Maryland

Michael A. Siegel, DDS, MS
Associate Professor
Department of Oral Medicine and
   Diagnostic Sciences
Dental School

Department of Dermatology
Medical School
University of Maryland at Baltimore
Baltimore, Maryland

Mohan Suntharalingam, MD
Assistant Professor and Vice Chairman
Department of Radiation Oncology
Medical School
University of Maryland at Baltimore
Baltimore, Maryland

Victoria A. Wilson, MSW, LCSW-C
Clinical Director
Medical Crisis Counseling Center
Department of Psychiatry
University of Maryland Medical Center
Baltimore, Maryland

Janet A. Yellowitz, DMD, MPH
Associate Professor
Director, Geriatric Dentistry
Baltimore College of Dental Surgery
Dental School
University of Maryland at Baltimore
Baltimore, Maryland

PART I

Diagnosis

CHAPTER 1

Epidemiology of Oral Cancer

Remy H. Blanchaert, Jr, MD, DDS

Cancer is the second leading cause of death in the United States. For 1999, the estimated number of new cancer cases was 1,221,800. The number of cancer-related deaths was expected to be 563,100. The predicted number of cancer cases involving the oral cavity and oral pharynx was 29,800. Oral and pharyngeal cancer account for fewer than 2% (approximately 8,100) of all cancer-related deaths and just over 2% of all new cancer diagnoses.[1]

The most common cancer involving the oral cavity is squamous cell carcinoma. The oral mucosa is subject to numerous insults, some of which are a result of personal habits. Tobacco use and alcohol consumption can result in irreparable genetic injury. Viral injury is a less well-defined, but increasingly studied mechanism of cellular injury leading to the development of cancer. The presence of the human papillomavirus has been reported as an initiating factor in the development of squamous cell carcinoma.[2] Whenever the body fails to eliminate cells permanently altered by these mechanisms or can no longer adequately suppress their replication, squamous cell carcinoma develops. Cancer of the oral cavity and oral pharynx also occurs in the minor salivary glands. The cause of these tumors remains unknown.

This chapter provides an understanding of the incidence, prevalence, and risk of oral and pharyngeal cancer. Sections describe the methods by which data are gathered and reported; the age at which oral and pharyngeal cancer is identified; and the impact of the development of second primary cancers, cigarette smoking, and alcohol abuse. The final section of this chapter gives epidemiologic data for a group of 200 patients in the Department of Oral and Maxillofacial Surgery at the University of Maryland. These data provide further understanding of the roles of dentistry and dental-related subspecialties in the diagnosis and management of oral cancer.

Statistic Data Collection and Reporting of Cancer

Comprehension of the myriad data reporting cancer statistics requires an understanding of the mechanism by which these data are generated. The United States does not have a national cancer registry; therefore, the exact number of cancer cases, cancer deaths, and exact staging, and patient age, sex, and race is unknown. The most useful available current data come from a complicated data manipulation process that correlates the results of a small data collection program and census data to achieve estimates of relevant nationwide numbers. These data are obtained in an intense but limited program involving 11 specific areas designed to be representative of the nation as a whole. The areas chosen include cities, geographic areas, and states. This program is known as the National Cancer Institute's Surveillance, Epidemiology, and End Results (SEER) program. Data from the US Bureau of the Census are used with the SEER data in complex mathematical calculations to derive relevant estimates.

Incidence

The incidence rate of a particular disease is the number of new cases divided by the number of people at risk per unit of time. For oral and pharyngeal carcinoma, the incidence rate in 1996 was estimated at 11.3 per 100,000. Incidence varies according to both race and gender.[3]

Population changes can significantly affect incidence rates. Oral and pharyngeal cancer predominately affect elderly persons. The age of the population studied is therefore critical in assessing changes in incidence rates of these cancers. To identify changes in cancer incidence rates, the SEER program reviews the most current incidence data and corrects it to an age-adjusted population equivalent to that of 1970.

Assessment of the available data in this manner indicates a decline in the incidence rate of oral and pharyngeal cancer from 11.3 to 10.0 per 100,000 in 1996.[3] This decline is evident only through evaluation of the age-adjusted data. In raw form, the incidence data show no difference. Age-adjusted data are particularly relevant to those involved in research or promoters of public awareness and prevention. In such fields, identifying trends or demonstrating effectiveness is extremely important. Without the adjustments made for changes in the population, a far greater alteration in raw data would be required to identify a change in incidence.

Significant race and gender differences exist in incidence rates of oral and pharyngeal cancer. An overall incidence rate of 10.0 per 100,000 in 1995 (age-adjusted to 1970 population) correlates with an incidence rate of 14.7 per 100,000 for men and an incidence rate of 6.0 per 100,000 for women. Differences in race incidence rates in 1995 were also apparent. The incidence rate for whites of both sexes was 9.8 per 100,000 and for blacks, 12.3 per 100,000. The highest incidence rate was found in black men (20.6 per 100,000) compared to that of white men (14.2 per 100,000).[3]

Prevalence

Prevalence describes a specific disease process in a defined population, or the total number of cases of a disease. It provides a quick look at or "snapshot" of the impact of a disease on a particular population. As such, prevalence does not account for the number of patients

Table 1-1	Impact of Oral and Pharyngeal Cancer According to Lifetime Risk in Men (%)*		
	All types	Oral and pharyngeal	Prostate
Risk of development	44.66	1.49	17.00
Risk of death	23.61	0.42	3.56
*Adapted from Ries et al.[3]			

Table 1-2	Impact of Oral and Pharyngeal Cancer According to Lifetime Risk in Women (%)*		
	All types	Oral and pharyngeal	Breast
Risk of development	38.03	0.74	14.24
Risk of death	20.53	0.24	3.43
*Adapted from Ries et al.[3]			

cured or the number for whom treatment failed. Because of its limitations in describing the outcome of therapy for a particular disease, prevalence is rarely reported in cancer-related studies. Despite this, when attempting to develop an overall impression of the significance of a disease for an at-risk population, prevalence provides useful information.

In 1998 it was estimated that 8,246,000 individuals in the United States were affected by cancer (3,409,000 men and 4,837,000 women). Cancer of the oral cavity and oral pharynx accounted for only a small portion of these cases, with a prevalence of 211,000 (132,000 men and 79,000 women), or 2.5% of all cancers.[3] For the sake of comparison it is relevant to look at the prevalence of the most common cancers in men and women. While breast cancer is the most prevalent (41%) malignancy in women, prostate cancer is the most prevalent (29%) in men.[3]

Comparison of the relative lifetime risk of the development of cancer at specific sites or death from specific cancers is a means by which investigators evaluate the impact of particular cancers. To understand the impact of cancer of the oral cavity and oral pharynx, the risk of its development and the lifetime risk of death from it can be compared to the overall risk of all cancers at all sites or to specific cancers. Lifetime risk is typically expressed in percentages (Tables 1-1 and 1-2).

The vast majority of oral and pharyngeal malignancies occur in elderly persons (Table 1-3). Significant race and gender differences exist in patient age at diagnosis of and death from disease (see Table 1-3). The development of cancer of the oral cavity and oral pharynx before age 45 is rare and accounted for 11.6% of all cases of such cancer reported for 1991 to 1995. Surprisingly, 21% of all cases are diagnosed in patients older than age 74.[3] The aging of the population guarantees that the rate of diagnosis in older patients will continue to increase. This is a significant factor in the management of these patients, who tend to have significant comorbidity, which can influence therapy significantly.

Table 1-3	Age at Diagnosis and Death According to Gender and Race*	
Parameter	Diagnosis	Death
Total	64	68
Women	67	71
Men	63	66
Blacks	57	60
Women	58	63
Men	56	59
Whites	65	69
Women	68	71
Men	64	67

*Adapted from Ries et al.[3]

Second Primary Cancers

The inciting factors responsible for the development of oral and pharyngeal squamous cell carcinoma have deleterious effects on all of the mucosa of the upper aerodigestive tract. Lung cancer and cancer of the esophagus are strongly correlated with a previous carcinoma of the oral cavity or pharynx. Second and even multiple cancers following therapy for the index lesion are common. In fact, improved therapy of the index lesion has failed to yield significant changes in the overall survival of patients with head and neck cancer, predominately because of the influence of additional malignancies. The actuarial incidence of second malignancies of the upper aerodigestive tract increases each year that a patient survives the index cancer.[4]

The role of tobacco products and alcohol in the development of second malignancies has been studied extensively. Slaughter and colleagues were the first to use the term *field cancerization* to explain the effects of carcinogens on the mucosa of the upper aerodigestive tract.[5] A single institution found that second primary cancers developed within 5 years of successful treatment of the index cancer in one third of patients with advanced stage (Stage III and Stage IV) squamous cell carcinoma of the oral cavity, pharynx, larynx, and hypopharynx.[6] A more recent study identified an overall 13.5% incidence of second primary malignancies in a prospective study of 127 patients with head and neck squamous cell carcinoma.[7] Lung tumors accounted for the majority (41%) of second primary cancers, with head and neck (35%) and esophageal (24%) malignancies making up the remainder. The majority of second tumors were identified because of symptoms (14 of 17). Therapy is often limited at diagnosis of the second cancer because of the effects of the therapy administered in treating the first malignancy. Surgery is often the only option for treatment because curative doses of radiation therapy can be administered only once. Likewise, complications of therapy and outcome are affected by the previous treatment.

Cigarette smoking

Ninety percent of patients in whom oral squamous cell carcinoma develops are smokers. Persons who smoke experience six times the relative risk of nonsmokers for the development of malignancy.[8] Rothman and Keller[9] reported a relative risk of 1.5 among nondrinking smokers. The risk was increased with heavy smoking to 2.4 times control.

Evidence exists that cigarette smoking may play a role in tumorigenesis through the specific mutation of the p53 suppressor gene. This gene transcribes a nuclear protein that is important in DNA repair, transcription, and replication.[10] Investigators have identified rates of p53 mutation in heavy smokers that are significantly higher than those for nonsmokers.[11] The effects of alcohol in conjunction with tobacco appear to be augmented.

Alcohol Abuse

Determining the exact influence of the use of alcohol is impossible. Several studies, however, have demonstrated a direct correlation. A synergistic effect between alcohol and tobacco products has been documented as well. An excellent review by Ogden and Wight[12] outlines the likely mechanisms and provides a thorough review of the literature in regard to the role of alcohol in the genesis of oral carcinoma. The authors cite three mechanisms by which alcohol can initiate cellular injury leading to carcinoma: metabolism of ethanol to the highly toxic substance acetaldehyde, increased permeability of cell membranes secondary to direct solvent effects, and disruption of normal cellular DNA repair. Additional systemic effects related to alcohol consumption may also play a role. Alteration of liver function in chronic alcoholics may decrease the detoxification of substances capable of cellular injury. Suppression of T cell function and cytotoxicity of killer cells is another example.

Ethanol is metabolized to acetaldehyde by alcohol dehydrogenase. The acetaldehyde is subsequently converted to acetate by aldehyde dehydrogenase. Both enzymes have been isolated in the oral cavity; however, the activity of the alcohol dehydrogenase seems to be greater than that of aldehyde dehydrogenase. This could result in accumulation of the cytotoxic acetaldehyde in oral tissues. Alcohol has the ability to dissolve the extracellular lipids present in the oral mucosa, thereby increasing its permeability. Animal studies have documented increased penetration of oral mucosa by tobacco-related carcinogens in the presence of alcohol. These data provide an explanation for the synergistic effect of alcohol and tobacco. Cellular growth studies in culture utilizing alcohol in the medium have demonstrated increases in abnormal DNA repair and increased chromosomal breakages.

The University of Maryland Experience

To provide an understanding of the role of dentistry in the diagnosis and management of oral cancer, the following data on 200 patients with squamous cell carcinoma of the oral cavity and pharynx are provided. The vast majority of these patients were identified by dentists and referred to oral surgery specialists for evaluation. The patients were subsequently referred to the University of Maryland for definitive care. These data were compiled from a consecutive sample of 200 patients from the University of Maryland Oral and Maxillofacial Surgery Database. These cases were reviewed retrospectively to identify relevant demographic data, staging, risk factors, and outcomes.

Of the 200 patients for whom records were reviewed, 121 were men and 79 were women. Three of the patients had simultaneous multiple primary cancers. The age distribution for the group was weighted in favor of those older than 60. A total of 117 patients were 60 years of age or older at the time of presentation. At the extremes, 22 were 80 years of age or older and 10 were less than 40 years of age.

The distribution of cases was divided nearly equally between early (Stage I and Stage II) and late (Stage III and Stage IV). Early stage disease was seen in 101 cancers and late stage disease in 102. Surgery was the sole treatment modality used in 105 patients. Therapy for 55 of the patients consisted of surgery and adjuvant radiation therapy. Two patients were treated with surgery, radiation therapy, and chemotherapy. The remainder of the patients received either radiation therapy alone or with chemotherapy.

Cigarette use was a contributing factor in 161 of the cases. A small group of 39 patients reported that they had never used tobacco products. The majority of patients had a history of significant alcohol exposure. Of the 200 patients, 164 were either current or previous drinkers, and the remaining 36 had little or no experience with alcohol.

At evaluation, reviewers were unable to follow up 32 patients (16%). No evidence of disease was present in 113 patients (56.5%). Death related to the index cancer was identified for 36 patients (18%). A second primary cancer had been identified in 30 patients (15%) and resulted in the death of 8 patients (4%).

Summary

Oral and pharyngeal cancer has a significant impact on the population in the United States. Early diagnosis of disease provides the best opportunity for effective therapy with an acceptable outcome. The dental community as a whole, and the general dentist in particular, is the first line of defense against the disease. A thorough examination of the oral cavity and oral pharynx should be completed in every dental patient. Timely referral of any suspicious lesion for evaluation and treatment is mandatory. Limitation of risk to smokers and drinkers alone will result in a failure to diagnose cancer in all patients. This is true for two reasons. First, not all malignancies of the oral cavity and pharynx are associated with identifiable risk factors. Second, despite the correlation of smoking and drinking with oral squamous cell carcinoma, oral cancer develops in a number of patients without these characteristic risk factors.

This chapter has defined the parameters by which the impact of oral and pharyngeal cancer is assessed. Relevant trends in the disease have been identified. The effects of tobacco and alcohol in the process of cellular injury leading to the development of oral cancer have been described, as have second primary cancers and their relation to outcome.

References

1. Landis SH, Murray T, Bolden S, Wingo PA. Cancer statistics, 1999. CA Cancer J Clin 1999;49:8.

2. Ostwald C, Muller P, Barten M, Rutsatz K, Sonnenburg M, Milde-Langosch K. Human papillomavirus DNA in oral squamous cell carcinoma and normal mucosa. J Oral Pathol Med 1994;23:220.

3. Ries LAG, Kosary CL, Hankey BF, et al. SEER Cancer Statistics Review, 1973–1995. Bethesda, MD: National Cancer Institute, 1998.

4. Batsakis JG. Syncronous and metacronous carcinomas in patients with head and neck cancer. Int J Radiat Oncol Biol Phys 1984;10:2163.

5. Slaughter DL, Southwick HW, Smejkal W. "Field cancerization" in oral stratified squamous epithelium: Clinical implications of multicenteric origin. Cancer 1953;6:963.

6. Vikram B, Strong EW, Shah JP, Spiro R. Second malignant neoplasms in patients successfully treated with multimodality treatment for advanced head and neck cancer. Head Neck Surg 1984;6:734.

7. Dhooge IJ, DeVos M, Van Cauwenberge PB. Multiple primary malignant tumors in patients with head and neck cancer: Results of a prospective study and future prospectives. Laryngoscope 1998;108:250.

8. Mashberg A, Bofetta P, Winkelman R, Garfinkel L. Tobacco smoking, alcohol drinking and cancer of the oral cavity and oropharynx among U.S. veterans. Cancer 1993;72:1369.

9. Rothman KJ, Keller AZ. The effect of joint exposure to alcohol and tobacco on the risk of cancer of the mouth and pharynx. J Chronic Dis 1972;25:711.

10. Levine AJ, Momand J, Finlay CA. The p53 tumor suppressor gene. Nature 1991;351:453.

11. Boyle JO, Hakim J, Koch W, van der Riet P, Hruban RH, Roa RA, et al. The incidence of p53 mutations increases with progression of head and neck cancer. Cancer Res 1993;53:447.

12. Ogden GR, Wight AJ. Aetiology of oral cancer: Alcohol. Br J Oral Maxillofac Surg 1998;36:247.

CHAPTER 2

Pathogenesis and Progression of Oral Cancer

John J. Sauk, DDS, MS, Mark A. Reynolds, DDS, PhD, and Ricardo Della Coletta, DDS, PhD

As indicated in chapter 1, oral and oropharyngeal squamous cell carcinomas represent only a small percentage, 2% to 3%, of the incidence of all cancers. The ratio of affected men to women recently has decreased from 3:1 to 2:1, primarily because of increased smoking by women. Despite what appear to be recent developments in the treatment of cancer, the survival rate of patients with oral and oropharyngeal cancer has remained discouragingly low. To reverse this trend, it is necessary to identify risk factors, such as identification of polymorphisms for enzymes metabolizing alcohol, and to detect clinical lesions early in their acceleration of clonal evolution.

Etiology of Oral Cancer

A number of factors contribute to the development of oral cancer; however, the use of all forms of tobacco and alcohol heads this list. Furthermore, there is considerable evidence that the time-dose relationship of carcinogens found in tobacco smoke as well as in the tobacco itself is of paramount importance in the cause of oral cancer.[1-5] For that reason, cigar and pipe smoking provide greater risk than cigarette smoking. Likewise, the use of various smokeless tobaccos in any form increases the risk for developing cancer especially of the gingival and buccal mucosa.

Alcohol consumption is also an important contributing factor to the development of oral cancer.[6-9] However, the mechanism by which alcohol consumption is implicated in this process is yet to be conclusively identified. Earlier studies implied that alcohol may irritate oral mucosa or serve as a solvent for carcinogens present in other sources. Furthermore, evidence is accumulating that ethanol and its metabolites, specifically acetaldehyde, appear to be directly responsible for the development of oral squamous cell carcinomas.[10,11] Although free-radical damage from these compounds or contaminants such as N-nitrosamines and urethane have been considered, perturbation of cell cultures has revealed that acetaldehyde—but not ethanol—results in the development of genetic instabilities.[12] These instabilities are likely the result of acetaldehyde forming adducts with DNA, since such adducts have been shown to initiate cellular transformation and inhibit DNA repair both in vitro and in vivo.[13,14]

Approximately 80% of ethanol is oxidized to acetaldehyde by alcohol dehydrogenase (ADH). There are several ADH subtypes with varying kinetic properties. Alcohol dehydrogenase type 3 is polymorphic in whites, and enzymes encoded by the ADH3[1] allele metabolize alcohol 2.5 times faster than the enzyme encoded by the ADH3[2] allele. As such, there is speculation that ADH3[1] genetic polymorphism may modify the risk of alcohol-related oral cancer.[10]

To support this theory, recent studies have shown that heavy drinkers possess a 40-fold increased risk of oral cancer compared to nondrinkers with the alcohol dehydrogenase type 3, ADH3[1–1] genotype. Moreover, the risk among heavy drinkers possessing the ADH3[1–1] genotype was 5.3 compared with the other ADH3 genotypes (ADH3[1–2], ADH3[2–2]). These risks were greater for tumors arising in the oral cavity than for tumors occurring in the pharynx. Although these data support the notion that ADH3[1–1] genotype substantially increases the risk of ethanol-related oral cancer and the carcinogenecity of acetaldehyde, further studies to include polymorphic ADH2 and cytochrome P450IIE1 genes, which encode other proteins that metabolize ethanol, should further define this relationship.[1] In addition to alcohol metabolites, products of the fungus *Candida albicans,* N-nitrobenzylmethylamine, has been implied as a possible carcinogen[15,16]; however, compelling evidence for this association has not been forthcoming.

The link between some viruses and some types and locations of oral cancer is evolving. Epstein-Barr virus has been linked to Burkitt's lymphoma and nasopharyngeal carcinoma where gene products of the virus appear to disrupt apoptosis.[17] Unlike other viral forms of oral cancer, Kaposi's sarcoma in early stages begins as an angiohyperplastic-inflammatory lesion mediated by inflammatory cytokines and angiogenic factors. This hyperproliferative state is triggered or amplified by infection with the Kaposi's sarcoma–associated herpesvirus (KSHV)/human herpesviruses type 8 (HHV8). The basis for such activation is that the genome of KSHV contains the open reading frames (ORFs) encoding for enzymes and viral structural proteins found in other herpesviruses. In addition, KSHV also contains an unprecedented number of ORFs pirated during viral evolution from cellular genes. These include proteins such as BCL-2 and cyclin homologues that alter growth; chemokine receptors, which induce angiogenesis; and CD21 and cytokine homologues that regulate antiviral immunity. Interestingly, the human immunodeficiency virus type 1 Tat protein appears to be responsible for the higher grade of aggressiveness of AIDS-associated Kaposi's sarcoma as compared to other forms of Kaposi's sarcoma.[18–22]

The human papillomavirus (HPV) subtypes 16 and 18 have been found in oral squamous cell carcinomas occurring primarily in the soft palate,[16,23] while verrucous carcinoma has been identified as a lesion related to HPV subtypes 11 and 16.[24] A mechanism by which HPV contributes to carcinogenesis is through the production of viral proteins E6 and E7, which form complexes with the tumor suppressor retinoblastoma gene (Rb gene) product and p53 that jeopardize DNA repair mechanisms and spur acceleration of the cell cycle.[25–28] Thus, it would appear that gene therapy directed at providing p53 by such modalities as recombinant adenovirus p53[29] might be of questionable utility in HPV-related cancers.[30] However, recombinant adenovirus p53 has been shown to suppress cervical cancer cells bearing HPV 18.[31] Nevertheless, the Rb gene is rarely affected in most forms of oral squamous cell carcinoma.[32]

Chronic irritation is generally regarded as a modifier rather than an initiator of oral cancer.[33] As such, the association of chronic inflammation with cancers has been coupled with the development of chronic diffuse epithelial hyperplasia, which is regarded as a common precursor to intraepithelial neoplasia. The basis for the latter view resides in the stimulation by growth factors and proliferation-inducing reactive oxygen species produced by lymphocytes and macrophages of chronic inflammatory infiltrates in the subepithelial stroma.[33-35]

In support of this notion, subepithelial inflammatory cells in gingiva have been shown to induce epidermal growth factor (EGF) and EGF receptors in the overlying squamous epithelium,[36] and the overexpression of EGF receptors is a common feature in oral cancer.[37,38] Examples of chronic inflammation associated with neoplasia include the aforementioned evolution of Kaposi's sarcoma from an angiohyperplastic inflammatory lesion, from the larynx where subepithelial inflammation is a predicator of progression to carcinoma,[36,39] and in respiratory mucosa where tobacco smoke induces stratified squamous metaplasia from which intraepithelial neoplasia emerges.[40] Although the importance of hyperproliferation to the development of cancer is still somewhat controversial, the balance of arguments is currently tipped toward this factor being a nonobligatory antecedent.[34,35,41]

Pathogenesis of Oral Cancer

Exposure of epithelial cells over time to carcinogens produces an increase in genomic aberrance due to unrepaired DNA breakage with secondary abnormal structural changes. The term *genomic instability* has been suggested to designate all types of perpetual and hereditary structural changes of all sizes of the genome resulting from such exposures. These changes or genomic structural variations (GSVs) are all-inclusive and range from point mutations to loss of myriad genes as part of a chromosome arm or even an entire chromosome.[33,42] Such GSVs have been shown to occur at a number of levels of DNA organization. Accordingly, GSVs may occur at the level of primary DNA sequence and encompass single nucleotides and oligonucleotide sequences within a gene, or they may include DNA segments containing many genes. In so doing, a DNA segment (amplicon) may exhibit a gain, loss, or recombination, even at the level of a whole chromosome, and thus display karyotypic distortion of chromosome structure and number.[33]

Genes whose expression is required to maintain the constancy of duplicating and segregating the genome have been designated as *genomic stability genes* (GSGs), and mutations in any of these genes lead to genomic instability.[33,42] Boone et al[33] have noted that the genomic instability produced by mutation of a genomic stability gene contributes to the risk of neoplasia; hence, these genes are likely considered to represent tumor suppressor genes. Correspondingly, GSGs control (1) products of genes that catalyze foraging of reactive oxygen species and carcinogens prior to their damaging DNA; (2) balanced nucleotide pools; (3) DNA replication and repair; (4) synthesis and coordination of cell division and DNA segregation; and (5) cell cycle check points impeding survival of cells with inordinate DNA damage.[33]

It is generally accepted that the exposure of oral mucosa to carcinogens (eg, tobacco smoke or acetaldehyde) takes place over a broad area, which increases the risk of hyperproliferation and gene damage. Accordingly, neoplastic clonal expansions may emerge at more than one site in epithelium that has developed strewn genomic instability due to persistent exposure to carcinogens. The multi-centric development of cancer, each progressing independently to carcinoma, was termed *field cancerization* by Slaughter et al.[43] In what is considered today a classic treatise, they describe observations of 783 patients in which multicentric in situ intraepithelial changes progressed independently to squamous cell carcinoma of the oral cavity.[43] Recently, Leong et al[44] have exploited this phenomenon by using microsatellite analysis to determine whether solitary squamous cell carcinomas in the lungs of patients with head and neck squamous cell carcinoma were manifesting another primary neoplasm or a metastatic tumor.

Since the publication of Slaughter et al, it has become clear that this progression to carcinoma occurs through clonal evolution, where perseverance within a cell population containing genomic structural variants undergoes clonal expansion more expeditiously than in surrounding cells.[45–47] The propensity for such clonal expansion appears to be especially true in those populations where genomic instability has resulted in dysregulation of apoptosis (ie, programmed cell death),[48] such as in the amplification of the amplicon 11q13 that includes cyclin D1.[49–52] Supplementary clonal expansion of aberrant cells may occur within the same primary expanding clone, or at other sites with independent lines of clonal evolution. Therefore, multiple clonal expansions may take place at different sites in the same tumor.[33,40,53]

The repercussion of clonal expansion is a ceaseless hastening of a cycle composed of an increased rate of production of neoplastic cells, genomic structural variants, and clonal variants. All of these cells and variants grow more rapidly, but are tempered by the increased production rate of cells undergoing apoptosis. The impetus of such cycles, as constraints for homeostasis disappear, is toward a selection to increasing disorder and heterogeneity.[1,6,33,40]

The finding of allelic loss of chromosome 9p in microscopically normal appearing hyperplastic epithelium adjacent to intraepithelial neoplastic lesions of the head and neck is an example of a predysplastic or premorphologic change associated with genomic instability.[47] An additional illustration is the demonstration, using chromosome-specific probes, of multiple clones with aneusomy/polysomy occurring in normal, nonhyperplastic epithelium adjacent to intraepithelial neoplasia of the head and neck.[54] However, with clonal expansion, the number and size of aneusomic clones increase with progression from normal nonhyperplastic to hyperplasia to dysplasia to cancer.[55] To support this idea, the genetic progression during intraepithelial neoplasia of head and neck squamous cell carcinoma, assessed with microsatellite analysis of allelic loss, has shown that the earliest losses are of 9p in squamous hyperplasia; followed by losses of 3p and 17p in dysplasia; then of 11q, 13q, and 14q in carcinoma in situ; and 5p and 4q after invasion (Fig 2-1).[47]

However, in a study of allelotypic differences in salivary gland neoplasms, Johns et al[56] discovered that salivary gland tumors display allelic loss patterns different from many other tumors, suggesting distinct genetic pathways and possible etiologies in the initiation and progression of these neoplasms. Pleomorphic adenomas demonstrated few areas of allelic loss; the most prominent chromosomal arm involved was 12q, lost in more than 35% of informative cases. The most significant allelic losses in adenoid cystic carcinoma were 1p, 2p, 6q, 17q, 20p, and 19q. Mucoepidermoid carcinoma showed 50% or greater loss at 2q, 5p, 12p, and 16q. As previously noted, losses at 9p, 3p, and 17p are common in squamous cell carcinoma of the head and neck; however, only the carcinoma ex-mixed tumors demonstrated loss at these loci, consistent with progression to a more aggressive phenotype.[56]

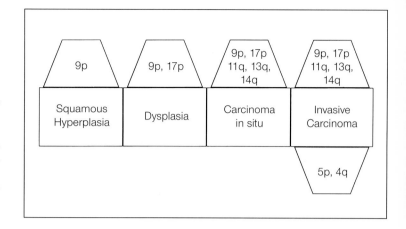

Fig 2-1 A graphic depiction of allelic loss detected within intraepithelial compartments in squamous hyperplasia, dysplasia, carcinoma in situ, and invasive carcinoma. Alleles depicted below the epithelial compartments signify changes specific to invasive disease.

Moreover, analyses in many laboratories of the allelotypes of many types of cancer, including oral squamous cell carcinoma, have shown that the frequency of allelic loss increases with time and tumor grade.[49,57–59]

Microsatellite analysis of oral lichen planus, a condition suggested by some to represent a preneoplastic condition, at nine loci frequently involved in oral squamous cell carcinoma revealed that loss of heterozygosity was detected only on a single chromosome arm. Furthermore, in this study such losses occurred on more than one chromosome in dysplasia and cancer, and the frequency of this multiple loss correlated significantly with increasing degrees of dysplasia and progression into squamous cell carcinoma. These data provide further evidence to support the notion that the proclivity of neoplastic cells possess an abnormal increase in phenotypic heterogeneity of structure and function.[60] Although these findings do not support oral lichen planus as a lesion at risk for malignant transformation, it does place these lesions in a category that correlates to conditions of reactive proliferation disorders and provides a mechanism for sustaining clonal expansion.

Neoplastic Progression

Neoplastic progression ensuing from initial clonal expansion, invasion of the basement membrane to culminate in a condition of extensive bulk, invasiveness, disseminated metastasis, and death has properties defined by both rate and extent.[33] Thus, the magnitude of neoplastic progression can be estimated from (1) the clinical level; (2) the tissue level, by assessing the breadth of invasion and nodal metastasis; (3) the cytonuclear level, as the degree of variation of nuclear size, shape, and especially chromatin texture; and (4) the molecular level, such as aneuploidy/aneusomy and the extent of microsatellite instability and frequency of allelic loss. Thus, the characteristic clinical properties of neoplastic progression, namely, the constant increase in cell proliferative rates, in genotypic and phenotypic heterogeneity,[60] and in total bulk and degree of dissemination, all derive from accelerating clonal evolution.

These considerations are becoming more apparent as the molecular basis of recognizing and predicting oral neoplasia is investigated.[33] For example, classically the morphologic progression of intraepithelial neoplasia is initially

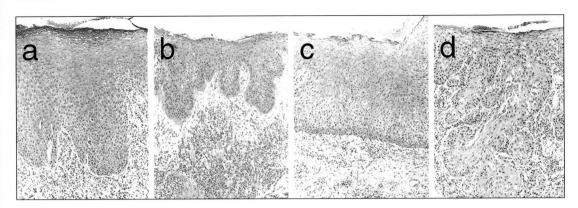

Fig 2-2 Development of intraepithelial neoplasia. (a) An example of epithelial hyper-plasia; (b) a mucosal section possessing features of dysplasia; (c) a mucosal biopsy revealing dysplasic changes extending to the surface as carcinoma in situ; (d) a spec-imen in which the dysplasia is accompanied by invasion of the tumor cells through the basement membrane into the underlying connective tissue.

characterized by pronounced basal cell hyper-plasia, usually with an irregular basement membrane profile, but without cytologic abnormalities. As previously noted, such find-ings in oral mucosa are generally associated with 9p allelic losses.[47] Progression to mild dysplasia includes the morphologic pattern previously described, but with cytologic abnormalities consisting of an increased nuclear cytoplasmic ratio, nuclear hyperchro-matism, and irregular nuclear chromatin which is confined to the basal layer (approxi-mately one third of the full thickness of the epithelium).

Moreover, progression to moderate dyspla-sia extends these changes to one half of the full thickness of the epithelium involved. The bottom portion of the spinous layer is disor-ganized, and there is a loss of normal layering or polarity. Occasionally, dyskeratotic cells may contain or be replaced by larger cells resembling those of the spinous layer. Such changes are coincident with allelic loss at 3q and 17q. Severe dysplasia or carcinoma in situ—demonstrating 11q, 13q, and 14q loss-es—taken as one category represent near full thickness involvement with no evidence of maturation. In severe dysplasia, dyskeratotic cells are more frequent, and the spinous layer is usually very disorganized and hard to iden-tify, although the surface may show some mat-uration. Invasive carcinoma is characterized by the cytologic changes previously described, with the hallmark being the escape of cells from the epithelial compartment through the basement membrane and allelic loss common-ly observed at 5p and 4q (Fig 2-2).[47] However, there is a strong trend to place greater weight on cytologic evidence of dysplasia than on the degree of involvement of the epithelial com-partment, because invasive carcinoma may emerge from dysplastic lesions involving less than half of the epithelial compartment.

In addition, amplified proto-oncogenes, or cellular oncogenes, have been found sporadi-cally in a broad spectrum of tumor types, whereas recurrent amplification of a particular gene or genomic region seems to be limited to a few tumor types.[61] Although an understand-ing of prevalence of amplification is still incomplete, this evolving field is providing a clearer picture of the neoplastic process and its progression. For example, amplification of genes in the 11q13 microsatellite has been found in head and neck cancers as well as a plethora of cancers in other body locations. Thus, 11q13 may be one of the most frequently amplified regions in human cancers.[62–64] Generally, such amplifications are only threefold to tenfold, raising a question about the significance of such augmentations. For example, in spite of the amplification of HSR1/FGF4 and INT2/FGF3, the expression of both fibroblastic growth factor 3 (FGF3) and fibroblastic growth factor 4 (FGF4) is low or undetectable. Although the basis for this is still not understood, it appears that FGF3 and FGF4 require the amplification of BCL1, which is thought to deregulate the nearby cyclin D1 gene (CYCD1).[61,65] As CYCD1 is immediately involved in regulating the G,S transition of the cell cycle, enhanced expression could perturb cell division and thereby contribute to tumorigenesis.[66] However, DNA amplified at 11q13 is extremely complex and harbors other amplified genes.[61]

For example, the EMS1 gene has been shown to be amplified in squamous cell carcinoma of the head and neck and associated with a more aggressive histologic composition, including cytologic grade and a diffusely infiltrative growth pattern.[67] The EMS1 gene product is designated as the human homologue of cortactin, which was initially identified as a substrate for the tyrosine kinase pp60v-src in chicken fibroblasts.[68] Furthermore, cortactin has been suggested as an important linker protein between membrane-bound receptors and the microfilament system. Interestingly, in both transformed cells and human squamous cell carcinomas, cortactin is relocated from the cytoplasm and accumulates to modified focal adhesion sites, which are believed to deregulate the cellular adhesive properties.[69]

Overexpression of EMS1/cortactin in NIH3T3 fibroblasts was shown to increase cell motility and invasion in vitro.[70] Recently, the CBP2 gene has been mapped to 11q13.5.[71] This gene codes for the protein Hsp47, which is a glycoprotein that binds specifically to collagen I, collagen IV, and gelatin. Hsp47 is also a resident endoplasmic reticulum protein closely associated with the production of procollagens.[72–76] However, like cortactin, Hsp47 may be redistributed to the cell membrane in some squamous cell carcinoma cell lines.[77] In addition, Hsp47 has been localized in lymph node metastases of some squamous cell carcinomas, suggesting that this protein may be a marker for malignancy.[78]

However, assessing the role of any of these genes in malignancy is complicated by discontinuities within the amplified DNA, likely due to secondary rearrangements.[33] Hence, although an amplified oncogene also may be present in a major proportion of cells of an individual tumor,[79] it is currently impossible to assign oncogene amplification a particular role in the multistep evolution of cancer cells.[61]

An important consideration regarding the pathogenesis and progression of oral cancer, particularly neoplasms derived from stratified squamous epithelium is the terminology used to describe various diagnostic features of intraepithelial lesions prior to invasion. Boone et al,[33] in a treatise on chemoprevention, make a strong argument that "terms such as severe atypia, dysplasia, and severe dysplasia describe epithelial cells that imperceptibly differ from the morphology of cells at the time of invasion." Although the onset of neoplastic disease appears approximately a decade before invasiveness, the notion that intraepithelial neoplasia described by these terms is fundamentally different from that of invasive cancer and requires "conversion" to become malignant is fallacious. Boone et al[33] reinforced the idea promulgated by Foulds[80] that such changes within the epithelial compartment are indicative of neoplasia. Furthermore, the term *carcinoma in situ,* given to indicate a higher risk of early invasion than the term *severe dysplasia,* is inaccurate: the cells underlying both of these diagnoses are essentially identical and form a single spectrum of neoplastic change.[33]

Summary

The development and progression of oral cancer have at least two antecedent controlling factors. The first is hyperproliferation, which may not be obligatory. The second and essential antecessor is the development of genetic instability, which is characterized by an increased rate of unrepaired DNA breaks and the formation of abnormal genomic structures. Oral cancer, like many other forms of cancer, is multifocal, demonstrating clonal evolution with intralesional generation of genomic structural variant cells and enhanced phenotypic heterogeneity. Ultimately, if treatment is delayed or left unchecked, these features lead to the progression of the cancer and culminate in death. Consequently, there is a special need for early diagnosis and the development of chemoprevention and gene therapy regimens prior to the establishment of intraepithelial neoplasia and most certainly to invasion.

References

1. Blot WJ, McLaughlin JK, Winn DM, Austin DF, Greenberg RS, Preston-Martin S, et al. Smoking and drinking in relation to oral and pharyngeal cancer. Cancer Res 1988;48:3282–3287.

2. Franceschi S, Talamini R, Barra S, Baron AE, Negri E, Bidoli E, et al. Smoking and drinking in relation to cancers of the oral cavity, pharynx, larynx, and esophagus in northern Italy. Cancer Res 1990;50:6502–6507.

3. Elwood JM, Pearson JC, Skippen DH, Jackson SM. Alcohol, smoking, social and occupational factors in the aetiology of cancer of the oral cavity, pharynx and larynx. Int J Cancer 1984;34:603–612.

4. Franco EL, Kowalski LP, Oliveira BV, Curado MP, Pereira RN, Silva ME, et al. Risk factors for oral cancer in Brazil: A case-control study. Int J Cancer 1989; 43:992–1000.

5. Xu J, Gimenez-Conti IB, Cunningham JE, Collet AM, Luna MA, Lanfranchi HE, et al. Alterations of p53, cyclin D1, Rb, and H-ras in human oral carcinomas related to tobacco use. Cancer 1998;83:204–212.

6. Talamini R, Franceschi S, Barra S, La Vecchia C. The role of alcohol in oral and pharyngeal cancer in non-smokers, and of tobacco in non-drinkers. Int J Cancer 1990;46:391–393.

7. Tuyns AJ, Esteve J, Raymond L, Berrino F, Benhamou E, Blanchet F, et al. Cancer of the larynx/hypopharynx, tobacco and alcohol: IARC international case-control study in Turin and Varese (Italy), Zaragoza and Navarra (Spain), Geneva (Switzerland) and Calvados (France). Int J Cancer 1988;41:483–491.

8. Kabat GC, Wynder EL. Type of alcoholic beverage and oral cancer. Int J Cancer 1989;43:190–194.

9. Martinez I. Factors associated with cancer of the esophagus, mouth, and pharynx in Puerto Rico. J Natl Cancer Inst 1969;42:1069–1094.

10. Harty LC, Caporaso NE, Hayes RB, Winn DM, Bravo-Otero E, Blot WJ, et al. Alcohol dehydrogenase 3 genotype and risk of oral cavity and pharyngeal cancers. J Natl Cancer Inst 1997;89:1698–1705.

11. Sciubba JJ. Oral leukoplakia. Crit Rev Oral Biol Med 1995;6:147–160.

12. Grafstrom RC, Dypbukt JM, Sundqvist K, Atzori L, Nielsen I, Curren RD, et al. Pathobiological effects of acetaldehyde in cultured human epithelial cells and fibroblasts. Carcinogenesis 1994;15:985–990.

13. Vaca CE, Fang JL, Schweda EK. Studies of the reaction of acetaldehyde with deoxynucleosides. Chem Biol Interact 1995;98:51–67.

14. Fang JL, Vaca CE. Development of a 32P-postlabelling method for the analysis of adducts arising through the reaction of acetaldehyde with 2′-deoxyguanosine-3′-monophosphate and DNA. Carcinogenesis 1995; 16:2177–2185.

15. O'Grady JF, Reade PC. Candida albicans as a promoter of oral mucosal neoplasia. Carcinogenesis 1992;13:783–786.

16. Steinberg BM, DiLorenzo TP. A possible role for human papillomaviruses in head and neck cancer. Cancer Metastasis Rev 1996;15:91–112.

17. DiGiuseppe JA, Wu TC, Zehnbauer BA, McDowell PR, Barletta JM, Ambinder RF, et al. Epstein-Barr virus and progression of non-Hodgkin's lymphoma to Ki-1- positive, anaplastic large cell phenotype. Mod Pathol 1995;8:553–559.

18. Samaniego F, Markham PD, Gendelman R, Watanabe Y, Kao V, Kowalski K, et al. Vascular endothelial growth factor and basic fibroblast growth factor present in Kaposi's sarcoma (KS) are induced by inflammatory cytokines and synergize to promote vascular permeability and KS lesion development. Am J Pathol 1998;152:1433–1443.

19. Hann SR, Eisenman RN. Proteins encoded by the human c-myc oncogene: Differential expression in neoplastic cells. Mol Cell Biol 1984;4:2486–2497.

20. Weiss RA, Whitby D, Talbot S, Kellam P, Boshoff C. Human herpesvirus type 8 and Kaposi's sarcoma. J Natl Cancer Inst Monogr 1998;51–54.

21. Boshoff C, Weiss RA. Kaposi's sarcoma-associated herpesvirus. Adv Cancer Res 1998;75:57–86.

22. Boshoff C. Kaposi's sarcoma. Coupling herpesvirus to angiogenesis. Nature 1998;391:24–25.

23. Balaram P, Nalinakumari KR, Abraham E, Balan A, Hareendran NK, Bernard HU, Chan SY. Human papillomaviruses in 91 oral cancers from Indian betel quid chewers—high prevalence and multiplicity of infections. Int J Cancer 1995;61:450–454.

24. Lubbe J, Kormann A, Adams V, Hassam S, Gratz KW, Panizzon RG, Burg G. HPV-11- and HPV-16-associated oral verrucous carcinoma. Dermatology 1996;192:217–221.

25. Iglesias M, Yen K, Gaiotti D, Hildesheim A, Stoler MH, Woodworth CD. Human papillomavirus type 16 E7 protein sensitizes cervical keratinocytes to apoptosis and release of interleukin-1alpha (in process citation). Oncogene 1998;17:1195–1205.

26. Rapp L, Chen JJ. The papillomavirus E6 proteins. Biochim Biophys Acta 1998;1378:F1–19.

27. Munirajan AK, Kannan K, Bhuvarahamurthy V, Ishida I, Fujinaga K, Tsuchida N, et al. The status of human papillomavirus and tumor suppressor genes p53 and p16 in carcinomas of uterine cervix from India. Gynecol Oncol 1998;69:205–209.

28. Kubbutat MH, Vousden KH. New HPV E6 binding proteins: Dangerous liaisons? Trends Microbiol 1998;6:173–175.

29. Liu TJ, Ahang WW, Taylor DL, Roth JA, Goepfert H, Clayman GL. Growth suppression of human head and neck cancer cells by the introduction of a wild-type p53 gene via a recombinant adenovirus. Cancer Res 1994;54:3662–3667.

30. Prabhu NS, Somasundaram K, Satyamoorthy K, Herlyn M, El-Deiry WS. p73beta, unlike p53, suppresses growth and induces apoptosis of human papillomavirus E6-expressing cells. Int J Oncol 1998;13:5–9.

31. Hamada K, Zhang WW, Alemany R, Wolf J, Roth JA, Mitchell MF. Growth inhibition of human cervical cancer cells with the recombinant adenovirus p53 in vitro. Gynecol Oncol 1996;60:373–379.

32. Matzow T, Boysen M, Kalantari M, Johansson B, Hagmar B. Low detection rate of HPV in oral and laryngeal carcinomas. Acta Oncol 1998;37:73–76.

33. Boone CW, Bacus JW, Bacus JV, Steele VE, Kelloff GJ. Properties of intraepithelial neoplasia relevant to the development of cancer chemopreventive agents. J Cell Biochem 1997;28-29(suppl):1–20.

34. Cohen SM, Ellwein LB. Genetic errors, cell proliferation, and carcinogenesis. Cancer Res 1991;51:6493–6505.

35. Cohen SM, Purtilo DT, Ellwein LB. Ideas in pathology. Pivotal role of increased cell proliferation in human carcinogenesis. Mod Pathol 1991;4:371–382.

36. Blackwell KE, Calcaterra TC, Fu YS. Laryngeal dysplasia: Epidemiology and treatment outcome. Ann Otol Rhinol Laryngol 1995;104:596–602.

37. Ke LD, Adler-Storthz K, Clayman GL, Yung AW, Chen Z. Differential expression of epidermal growth factor receptor in human head and neck cancers. Head Neck 1998;20:320–327.

38. Kusukawa J, Harada H, Shima I, Sasaguri Y, Kameyama T, Morimatsu M. The significance of epidermal growth factor receptor and matrix metalloproteinase-3 in squamous cell carcinoma of the oral cavity. Eur J Cancer B Oral Oncol 1996;32B:217–221.

39. Blackwell KE, Fu YS, Calcaterra TC. Laryngeal dysplasia. A clinicopathologic study. Cancer 1995;75:457–463.

40. Boone CW, Kelloff GJ, Steele VE. Natural history of intraepithelial neoplasia in humans with implications for cancer chemoprevention strategy. Cancer Res 1992;52:1651–1659.

41. Farber E. Cell proliferation as a major risk factor for cancer: A concept of doubtful validity. Cancer Res 1995;55:3759–3762.

42. Cheng KC, Loeb LA. Genomic instability and tumor progression: Mechanistic considerations. Adv Cancer Res 1993;60:121–156.

43. Slaughter DP, Southwick HW, Smejkal W. Field cancerization in oral stratified squamous epithelium: Clinical implications of multicentric origin. Cancer 1951;6:963–968.

44. Leong PP, Rezai B, Koch WM, Reed A, Eisele D, Lee DJ, et al. Distinguishing second primary tumors from lung metastases in patients with head and neck squamous cell carcinoma. J Natl Cancer Inst 1998;90:972–977.

45. Scholes AG, Woolgar JA, Boyle MA, Brown JS, Vaughan ED, Hart CA, et al. Synchronous oral carcinomas: Independent or common clonal origin? Cancer Res 1998;58:2003–2006.

46. Cense HA, van Lanschot JJ, Fockens P, Obertop H, Offerhaus GJ. A patient with seven primary tumors of the upper aerodigestive tract: The process of field cancerization versus distant monoclonal expansion. Dis Esophagus 1997;10:139–142.

47. Califano J, van der Riet P, Westra W, Nawroz H, Clayman G, Piantadosi S, et al. Genetic progression model for head and neck cancer: Implications for field cancerization. Cancer Res 1996;56:2488–2492.

48. Lydiatt WM, Anderson PE, Bazzana T, Casale M, Hughes CJ, Huvos AG, et al. Molecular support for field cancerization in the head and neck. Cancer 1998;82:1376–1380.

49. Muller D, Millon R, Velten M, Bronner G, Jung G, Engelmann A, et al. Amplification of 11q13 DNA markers in head and neck squamous cell carcinomas: Correlation with clinical outcome. Eur J Cancer 1997;33:2203–2210.

50. Michalides RJ, van Veelen NM, Kristel PM, Hart AA, Loftus BM, Hilgers FJ, et al. Overexpression of cyclin D1 indicates a poor prognosis in squamous cell carcinoma of the head and neck. Arch Otolaryngol Head Neck Surg 1997;123:497–502.

51. Akervall JA, Michalides RJ, Mineta H, Balm A, Borg A, Dictor MR, et al. Amplification of cyclin D1 in squamous cell carcinoma of the head and neck and the prognostic value of chromosomal abnormalities and cyclin D1 overexpression. Cancer 1997;79:380–389.

52. Kyomoto R, Kumazawa H, Toda Y, Sakaida N, Okamura A, Iwanaga M., et al. Cyclin-D1-gene amplification is a more potent prognostic factor than its protein over-expression in human head-and-neck squamous-cell carcinoma. Int J Cancer 1997;74:576–581.

53. Wolff E, Girod S, Liehr T, Vorderwulbecke U, Ries J, Steininger H, et al. Oral squamous cell carcinomas are characterized by a rather uniform pattern of genomic imbalances detected by comparative genomic hybridisation. Oral Oncol 1998;34:186–190.

54. Voravud N, Shin DM, Ro JY, Lee JS, Hong WK, Hittelman WN. Increased polysomies of chromosomes 7 and 17 during head and neck multistage tumorigenesis. Cancer Res 1993;53:2874–2883.

55. Voravud N, Charuruks N, Mutirangura A. Squamous cell carcinoma of head and neck. J Med Assoc Thai 1997;80:207–218.

56. Johns MM, Westra WH, Califano JA, Eisele D, Koch WM, Sidransky D. Allelotype of salivary gland tumors. Cancer Res 1996;56:1151–1154.

57. Jin Y, Hoglund M, Jin C, Martins C, Wennerberg J, Akervall J, et al. FISH characterization of head and neck carcinomas reveals that amplification of band 11q13 is associated with deletion of distal 11q. Genes Chromosom Cancer 1998;22:312–320.

58. Gebhart E, Liehr T, Wolff E, Ries J, Fiedler W, Steininger H, et al. Pattern of genomic imbalances in oral squamous cell carcinomas with and without an increased copy number of 11q13. Int J Oncol 1998;12:1151–1155.

59. Meredith SD, Levine PA, Burns JA, Gaffey MJ, Boyd JC, Weiss LM, et al. Chromosome 11q13 amplification in head and neck squamous cell carcinoma. Association with poor prognosis. Arch Otolaryngol Head Neck Surg 1995;121:790–794.

60. Ames BN, Gold LS, Willett WC. The causes and prevention of cancer. Proc Natl Acad Sci USA 1995;92;5258–5265.

61. Schwab M. Amplification of oncogenes in human cancer cells. Bioessays 1998;20:473–479.

62. Gaudray P, Szepetowski P, Escot C, Birnbaum D, Theillet C. DNA amplification at 11q13 in human cancer: From complexity to perplexity. Mutat Res 1992;276:317–328.

63. Roelofs H, Schuuring E, Wiegant J, Michalides R, Giphart-Gassler M. Amplification of the 11q13 region in human carcinoma cell lines: A mechanistic view. Genes Chromosom Cancer 1993;7:74–84.

64. Lammie GA, Fantl V, Smith R, Schuuring E, Brookes S, Michalides R, et al. D11S287, a putative oncogene on chromosome 11q13, is amplified and expressed in squamous cell and mammary carcinomas and linked to BCL-1. Oncogene 1991;6:439–444.

65. Ames BN, Gold LS. Chemical carcinogenesis: Too many rodent carcinogens. Proc Natl Acad Sci USA 1990;87:7772–7776.

66. Hunter T, Pines J. Cyclins and cancer. Cell 1991;66:1071–1074.

67. Hui R, Campbell DH, Lee CS, McCaul K, Horsfall DJ, Musgrove EA, et al. EMS1 amplification can occur independently of CCND1 or INT-2 amplification at 11q13 and may identify different phenotypes in primary breast cancer. Oncogene 1997;15:1617–1623.

68. Schuuring E, Verhoeven E, Mooi WJ, Michalides RJ. Identification and cloning of two overexpressed genes, U21B31/PRAD1 and EMS1, within the amplified chromosome 11q13 region in human carcinomas. Oncogene 1992;7:355–361.

69. van Damme H, Brok H, Schuuring-Scholtes E, Schuuring E. The redistribution of cortactin into cell-matrix contact sites in human carcinoma cells with 11q13 amplification is associated with both overexpression and post-translational modification. J Biol Chem 1997;272:7374–7380.

70. Patel AS, Schechter GL, Wasilenko WJ, Somers KD. Overexpression of EMS1/cortactin in NIH3T3 fibroblasts causes increased cell motility and invasion in vitro. Oncogene 1998;16:3227–3232.

71. Ikegawa S, Nakamura Y. Structure of the gene encoding human colligin-2 (CBP2). Gene 1997;194:301–303.

72. Sauk JJ, Norris K, Hebert C, Ordonez J, Reynolds M. Hsp47 binds to the KDEL receptor and cell surface expression is modulated by cytoplasmic and endosomal pH. Connect Tissue Res 1998;37:105–119.

73. Nagata K. Expression and function of heat shock protein 47: A collagen-specific molecular chaperone in the endoplasmic reticulum. Matrix Biol 1998;16:379–386.

74. Nagata K, Hosokawa N. Regulation and function of collagen-specific molecular chaperone, HSP47. Cell Struct Funct 1996;21:425–430.

75. Hu G, Gura T, Sabsay B, Sauk J, Dixit SN, Veis A. Endoplasmic reticulum protein Hsp47 binds specifically to the N-terminal globular domain of the aminopropeptide of the procollagen I alpha 1 (I)-chain. J Cell Biochem 1995;59:350–367.

76. Sauk JJ, Smith T, Norris K, Ferreira L. Hsp47 and the translation-translocation machinery cooperate in the production of alpha 1(I) chains of type I procollagen. J Biol Chem 1994;269:3941–3946.

77. Hebert C, Norris K, Della-Coletta R, Reynolds M, Ordonez J, Sauk JJ. Cell surface colligin/hsp47 associates with tetraspanin protein CD9 in epidermoid carcinoma cell lines. J Cell Biochem (in press).

78. Morino M, Tsuzuki T, Ishikawa Y, Shirakami T, Yoshimura M, Kiyosuke Y, et al. Specific expression of HSP47 in human tumor cell lines in vitro. In Vivo 1997;11:17–21.

79. Schwab M, Ellison J, Busch M, Rosenau W, Varmus HE, Bishop JM. Enhanced expression of the human gene N-myc consequent to amplification of DNA may contribute to malignant progression of neuroblastoma. Proc Natl Acad Sci USA 1984;81:4940–4944.

80. Foulds L. Neoplastic Development. New York: Academic Press, 1969.

CHAPTER 3

The Oral Cancer Examination

Janet A. Yellowitz, DMD, MPH

There is hardly an oral lesion that at one stage or another cannot assume the same overt appearance as a squamous cell carcinoma—hence the concept of oral cancer as "the great mimicker."[1] The detection of oral cancer at an early state, when it is most amenable to treatment, is an important goal for the dental profession. Too often squamous cell carcinomas are dismissed as innocuous, benign ulcers, traumatic lesions, or soft tissue aberrations.

Each year in the United States, nearly 30,000 new cases of oral cancer are detected, with almost 9,000 deaths as a result of this disease. Almost all (90%) oral cancers are squamous cell carcinomas, which begin as surface lesions. Logically, it would seem that such surface lesions would be detected at an early stage; however, most oral cancers are diagnosed at a late stage of development. Most oral carcinomas are detected only after becoming symptomatic or invasive or after having metastasized to the cervical lymph nodes.[2] Once the patient experiences symptoms, squamous cell carcinomas are not difficult to diagnose; however, the detection and diagnosis of the early asymptomatic lesion presents a major challenge to the practitioner.

Diagnosis of Early Stage Oral Carcinomas

With the exception of malignant lesions of the skin, no cancers are more accessible to diagnosis than oral cancers.[3] Although most oral carcinomas occur at sites that lend themselves to direct examination and are well suited for detection,[4] the clinical presentation of early stage lesions differs markedly from advanced cancers.[5] Because early lesions have a highly variable presentation and do not exhibit the dramatic clinical changes associated with malignancy, they are often misdiagnosed.[5] To add to the difficulty of diagnosis, patients with early stage carcinomas do not present with pain or other symptoms. Thus, detecting an oral carcinoma is primarily dependent upon the clinician providing a comprehensive oral cancer examination and having a high level of suspicion and a willingness to ascertain the etiology of a lesion. It is important for the clinician to include oral carcinoma in the differential diagnosis of a multitude of ill-defined, variable-appearing lesions found in the oral cavity. The process of diagnosing asymptomatic lesions is often one of exclusion.

Early stage oral cancers have numerous and variable clinical appearances. Early lesions can appear as subtle, asymptomatic areas with superficial surface color and textural changes. They can appear as red, red-white speckled, or white lesions; areas of induration or ulceration; or infiltrative tumors. Early stage lesions can be hidden in the folds of mucosa at the base of the tongue. Soft tissue changes may appear to be the result of physical, chemical, or thermal trauma, or they may resemble or coexist with common entities such as candidiasis or lichen planus. Any nonhealing mucosal lesion, especially, although not exclusively, in a cancer predilection site, must be considered suspicious unless proven otherwise. Cancer predilection sites include the floor of the mouth, ventral and lateral borders of the tongue, retromolar trigone, and the soft palate/tonsillar complex.[6,7] The lower lip is the only site that has demonstrated a significant reduction in cancer incidence during the past few decades, likely due to the increased use of sunscreens.

The primary risk factors for oral cancer are current or previous use of tobacco products and/or alcohol consumption, exposure to sunlight (specifically for lip cancers), and being 40 years of age or older. The majority (75%) of squamous cell carcinomas have been associated with tobacco and alcohol use, and these habits increase the risk of oral carcinoma from 3 to 15 times that of the general population.[8] Individuals with a prior oral cancer are at highest risk for developing a second lesion.[9] Diet and nutrition have recently been identified as having a protective role against oral cancer.[10] Contrary to many practitioners' belief, chronic denture irritation has not been documented as a risk factor for oral cancer. However, risk factors alone do not predict who will be an oral cancer victim. Oral cancers develop in many patients with no risk factors. In a recent 5-year review of patients with oral cancer treated in a metropolitan hospital, 20% reported not using tobacco products and 21% reported not using alcohol.[11]

Like most cancers, oral cancer is a disease of older age. The average age at time of diagnosis is 60 years, and almost 95% of oral cancers occur in persons 40 years of age and older.[12] This fact is particularly important given the dramatic growth in the size of the population 50 years and older. The higher incidence of oral cancer associated with increasing age suggests that a time factor, involving the biochemical and biophysical processes of aging cells, may be in operation.[12]

As "physicians of the mouth," dentists are trained to detect an oral neoplasm while it is asymptomatic and innocuous. Given the easy access of the oral cavity, clinicians need to be able to recognize abnormalities that may indicate malignancy, as well as precancerous changes. Because oral cancer generally develops over an extended period, it is possible, as well as preferable, to detect incipient surface alterations characteristic of premalignancy in advance of actual invasive disease.[13,14] An oral cancer examination needs to be part of the oral evaluation of all patients. However, some dentists fail to provide a complete examination for every patient, while others have been found remiss in the detection and referral of oral cancer lesions for treatment.[15–17] Similarly, some clinicians are not familiar with the differential diagnosis of signs and symptoms, are not suspicious of lesions, or treat lesions empirically.[12] It has been hypothesized that practitioners do not detect early stage oral lesions because of their low level of suspicion of soft tissue changes, their tendency to focus on patient symptoms,[18] and their knowledge and attitudes related to oral cancer.[19,20]

Delay in Diagnosis

Oral cancer has been referred to as "the forgotten disease" and is frequently held in low priority by both health care providers and the public.[21] Delays in diagnosis have been related to the patient, the clinician, or both.[22] Delays in diagnosis lead to delays in treatment, to local extension of the lesion, to an increased risk for metastatic spread, and ultimately to a poorer outcome.

Diagnosing oral cancers at an early stage is critical to improving the survival rate and reducing the morbidity associated with this disease.[23] Recent studies have found that at the time of the oral cancer diagnosis, 36% of patients have localized disease, and 64% have regional, distant, or unstaged disease.[24] The 5-year survival rate for individuals initially presenting with localized disease is 81%, dramatically better than 42% for regional involvement and 17% for distant metastasis.[24] Thus it appears that the earlier the diagnosis and treatment, the better the patient's chances are for survival. Despite advances in therapy, little improvement in survival rates has been seen during the past several decades, primarily because most oral cancers are diagnosed when function is impaired, when the patient complains of symptoms, or when the lesions measure over 2 cm.[25]

Studies have found that the reason dentists do not detect oral lesions in their early stages is due to their knowledge, opinions, and practices related to oral cancer.[19,26–30] In a recent national survey, almost all dentists (98%) agreed that patients 40 years or older should have an oral cancer examination annually, yet 30% do not provide one during the patient's initial visit, and 41% do not examine these patients at recall visits.[31] Similarly, the study found that 20% of dentists do not provide oral cancer examinations for edentulous patients.[31] Since many edentulous patients do not seek oral health care

services on a routine basis,[32] this omission can have serious consequences. In addition, other studies have reported that dentists failed to recognize oral cancer in the majority (69%) of the cases presented to them,[16] and missed almost twice as many asymptomatic oral cancer cases as they found.[17] Another study reported that "professional delay" was significant in cases involving women, older persons, and small tumors.[33] Despite numerous efforts to increase the clinician's level of suspicion, this deficiency has persisted for more than 25 years.[34]

In general, people are more likely to visit a physician than a dentist. However, physicians are less likely than dentists to provide an oral cancer examination,[20,23] do not routinely check their patients to identify suspicious oral lesions,[35–38] and are less likely to refer lesions at an early stage.[27] This may be due to the fact that physicians have limited training in the oral cavity and oral cancer, and when they do examine the head and neck and find malignancies, they are likely to confuse them with traumatic, inflammatory, and infectious lesions.[39] Delay in diagnosis may also be due to a physician's belief that dentists are primarily responsible for detecting oral cancers.[15] Most physicians do not routinely ask their patients when they last received an oral examination or treatment from a dental professional. Only 3% of internal medicine residents documented having completed an oral cancer screening examination on their patients at high risk for oral cancer.[40]

Patients are also responsible for delaying the diagnosis of an oral cancer. A recent study found that more than one third of patients with oral cancer delayed seeking professional advice for more than 3 months after first being aware of a lesion.[41] In addition, patients tend to seek the care of a physician when experiencing symptoms of oral cancer. Jovanovic et al[42] found that the majority of patients with oral cancer consulted their family doctor prior to consulting other health care workers. In that study, the mean patient delay was 103 days, while the mean physician delay was 22 days. Prout et al[36] reported that 94% of patients presenting with oral cancer had made an average of 10.7 visits with medical care providers during the 2 years prior to their diagnosis, thus representing many missed opportunities for early detection. Studies have reported, and dentists have agreed, that patients are not knowledgeable about the risk factors, signs, or symptoms of oral cancer.[43] Without accurate information, people cannot be expected to make informed decisions about their own health, including the need for oral cancer examinations. Thus, programs are needed to educate the public about the signs and symptoms of oral cancer.

Detection of Oral Cancer

In a national survey of general dentists,[31] the majority reported their knowledge of oral cancer to be current and their training adequate to provide an oral cancer examination. Yet, over half of the dentists incorrectly identified "asymptomatic" as the most frequent patient complaint associated with early stage oral cancer, and 34% did not recognize early detection as a means of reducing morbidity and mortality from this disease. Almost two thirds (66%) of these dentists reported not palpating patients' cervical lymph nodes; thus they did not provide one of the primary components of an oral cancer examination. Since most practitioners spend the majority of their time treating the dentition and periodontal conditions, pathologic lesions of the soft tissue are often overlooked. Patients treated in dental practices that do not provide comprehensive oral cancer examinations are at an increased risk of not having an oral lesion diagnosed or of having the lesion diagnosed at an advanced stage.

Providing a thorough physical examination of the head, neck, and oral cavity is essential for all dentists and any clinician involved in detecting, diagnosing, and treating oral disease. The examiner assesses for the presence or absence of palpable adenopathy; the number, location, and size of palpable lymph nodes; and the clinical manifestation of disease, such as fixation of soft tissue or overlying skin, or paralysis of cranial nerves.[44] This examination provides critical information for the development of an appropriate differential diagnosis.

Because many oral cancers arise in apparently normal mucosa, it is important to assess all tissues carefully.[34] For some patients with oral cancer, the primary tumor may be easily identified because of its size and location, whereas other lesions may only be detected with a thorough head and neck examination. With prompt and decisive action, a clinician can save lives and reduce the morbidity associated with oral cancer. Conversely, inadequate diagnostic skill and improper examination technique can delay diagnosis and worsen the patient's prognosis.[45]

Components of the Oral Cancer Examination

A comprehensive oral cancer examination requires a review of the patient's medical and dental history; visual assessment of the head, neck, and oral cavity; and manual palpation of the regional cervical lymph nodes.[46]

Health history

Well-prepared medical and dental histories provide information pertinent to the etiology of oral conditions and aid in the identification of conditions that may increase the risk of disease.[47] Because smoking tobacco products and drinking alcohol have been shown to contribute to about 75% of oral cancers in the United States,[48] it is vital for the practitioner to be informed of the patient's use and history of use of these products. Recent studies have found that dentists either do not assess or are unaware of their patients' high-risk behaviors.[15,20] One study reported that while 71% of dentists assess their patients' previous tobacco use, only 36% assess alcohol use. Similarly, another study reported that dentists were less aware of their patients' tobacco habits (64%) and alcohol habits (40%) than were physicians.[15] Studies of health history forms used in dental and dental hygiene schools were found to be deficient in determining a patient's risk behaviors associated with oral cancer.[49,50] Without this information, providers can easily underassess a patient's risk for oral cancer, especially for those patients who only recently stopped using tobacco products or drinking alcohol.[51] However, absence of these factors does not preclude the need for all individuals to undergo a thorough oral cancer examination.

Visual assessment

Direct visualization of the mucosal surfaces is vital in detecting early lesions, which usually have little mass and minimal depth.[5] To optimize the clinician's ability to identify surface changes, the mucosal surfaces need to be dry and viewed under good illumination. Visualization prior to palpation improves the practitioner's ability to detect soft tissue changes.

Palpation

Palpation is particularly significant for the detection of primary lesions that are not read-ily visible. A lesion that appears superficial may be found upon palpation to be infiltrative and deep, suggesting a more extensive tumor. The presence of a metastatic lymph node in the neck can draw attention to a potential primary site.[52] Because one of the most important prognostic factors in patients with oral cancer is the status of the cervical lymph nodes,[52] palpation of the neck is essential for a complete oral examination.

Types of palpation

Gloved hands should be used to move or press tissues to detect changes in consistency and size. Using the pads of the index and middle fingers, moderate pressure should be used to move fingers over the underlying tissues in each area. Table 3-1 describes the types of palpation.

Palpation findings

A normal cervical lymph node is not palpable on routine examination. However, small, mobile, discrete, nontender nodes are frequently found in healthy people.[53] Palpable nodes are the primary sign of past or current lymph node disease and may indicate one of a large number of infectious, immune, or neoplastic diseases. In general, tender, soft, enlarged, and freely movable nodes suggest acute infection. Enlarged or tender nodes, if unexplained, call for a reexamination and a careful assessment of the cervical lymph nodes to distinguish between regional and generalized lymphadenopathy. Hard, nontender, fixed nodes may suggest a chronic infection or malignancy (Table 3-2).

Cervical lymph nodes

Head and neck cancers metastasize to the lymph nodes in the neck in a sequential, predictable pattern.[54] The lymphatics draining

Table 3-1   Types of Palpation

Type	Method	Example
Digital	Use of a single finger	Index finger applied to inner border of the mandible beneath the canine premolar area to determine the presence of tori or swellings.
Bidigital	Use of finger and thumb of the same hand	Palpation of the lips and cheeks.
Bimanual	Use of finger or fingers and thumb from each hand simultaneously	Index finger of one hand palpates the floor of the mouth intraorally, while finger or fingers of the other hand press on the same area extraorally from under the chin.
Bilateral	Both hands used at the same time to examine corresponding structures on opposite sides of the body	Fingers placed beneath chin to palpate submandibular lymph nodes. Comparisons between sides can be made. Useful technique to differentiate anatomic structures and unilateral variations.

Table 3-2   Guidelines for Lymph Node Palpation Characteristics

Hard or soft	Tender or nontender	Fixed or movable	Etiology
Soft	Tender	Movable	Acute infection or inflammation
Hard (or fixed)	Nontender	Movable or fixed	Malignancy or chronic infection

most primary sites in the head and neck are located in specific anatomic locations. During the examination, the clinician needs to be familiar with oral structures to differentiate changes in size, color, texture, and symmetry. For example, superficial cervical nodes can be palpated with relative ease by manipulation of the relaxed sternocleidomastoid muscle. Knowledge of the lymph node drainage patterns aids in locating the primary lesion (Fig 3-1). To provide health care professionals with common terminology, the regional lymph nodes of the head and neck are described by levels (Fig 3-2 and Table 3-3).

Examination Procedure

In the absence of definitive criteria to identify those most likely to have an oral carcinoma, annual oral cancer examinations are recommended for all patients. Combining the oral cancer examination with customary examination techniques, whether medical or dental, ensures its completion during the patient's initial and recall visits.

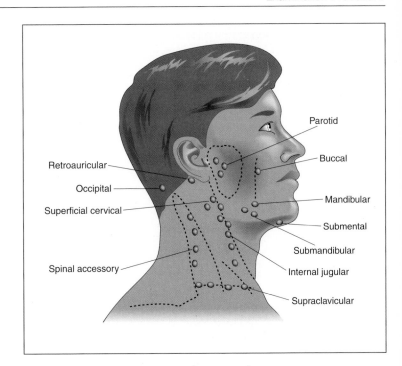

Parotid

Buccal

Retroauricular

Occipital

Superficial cervical

Mandibular

Submental

Submandibular

Spinal accessory

Internal jugular

Supraclavicular

Fig 3-1 Schematic diagram of lymph node location in head and neck (does not include all nodes).

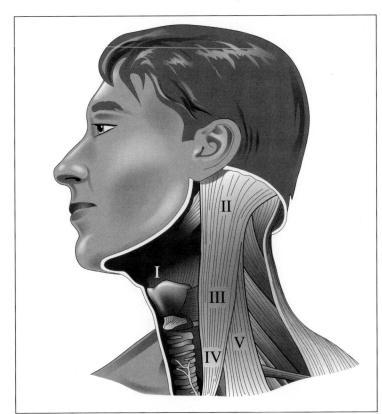

Fig 3-2 Schematic diagram of levels of lymph nodes found in neck. See Table 3-3 for anatomic boundaries.

Table 3-3	Lymph Nodes in the Neck	
Level	Nodes	Anatomic boundaries
I	Submandibular gland, submental nodes, auricular nodes (pre- and post-)	The submental triangle is formed by the midline anteriorly, the digastric muscle posteriorly, and the hyoid bone inferiorly; the submandibular triangle is bounded by the mandible and the digastric muscle.
II	Occipital nodes, jugular nodes, upper posterior cervical	Jugular nodes extend from the subdigastric area down to the carotid artery bifurcation; the upper posterior cervical triangle is above the entrance of the spinal accessory nerve.
III	Jugular nodes	Along the jugular vein between the carotid artery and its bifurcation; the posterior border of the sternocleidomastoid and omohyoid muscles.
IV	Jugular nodes, cervical chain	Below the omohyoid muscle; above the clavicle and between the carotid artery anteriorly and the omohyoid muscle posteriorly.
V	Middle posterior cervical, lower posterior cervical, supraclavicular	Formed by the posterior part of the sternocleidomastoid muscle, the trapezius muscle, and the posterior belly of the omohyoid muscle.

Sequence of procedures

Although the order of the examination procedures is a matter of individual choice, the clinician needs to establish a systematic routine to ensure that no area is overlooked. Using a step-by-step protocol helps to increase efficiency, conserve time, and maintain a professional atmosphere.[55] Thus, a clinician needs to select the protocol that best suits his or her work style.

Following a review of the patient's medical and dental history, the clinician should ask if the patient is experiencing discomfort in any areas of the mouth or neck. To reduce patient anxiety and concern, an explanation of what is being done and the reasons for the examination should be given to the patient. This is also an excellent time to educate the patient about the importance of routine oral examinations as well as the importance of self-examination to detect unusual changes. At a minimum,

patients need to be instructed to bring to their dentist's attention any lumps or bumps, painful areas, or changes in color, anatomy, or tissue texture, especially any change present for 14 days or longer. All findings should be recorded in the patient's chart.

The clinician begins with an overall appraisal of the patient:

• The patient should be seated comfortably with the head stabilized by a headrest cushion.
• The patient should remove eyeglasses and dental prostheses prior to the examination.
• The clinician should face the patient.
• Clean gloves should be worn and changed when moving from extraoral to intraoral examination.

Figure 3-3 lists the steps of a comprehensive oral cancer examination in a recommended, sequential order.

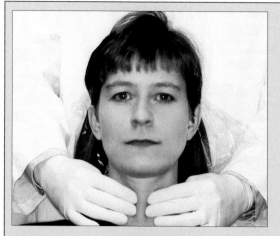

Anatomic location: Thyroid gland.*

Method: Have the patient face forward, leaning slightly forward to keep head and neck tissues relaxed. In anterior lower neck, locate the area just below the thyroid prominence (Adam's apple). Place fingers on one side of the trachea and gently push the thyroid gland toward the other side of the neck. With the other hand, exert circular digital compression on the gland. Have the patient swallow and feel the gland rise and fall. Alternatively, palpate the gland from behind the patient. Place fingers of both hands on the neck so the index fingers are just below the cricoid.

Warning signs: Masses, enlargements, nodules, asymmetries, tenderness.

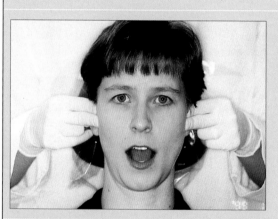

Anatomic location: Temporomandibular joint.

Method: Bilaterally place fingers of each hand just anterior to the outer meatus (tragus) of ears. Have the patient open and close the mouth several times and, while the jaw is open, move it from side to side and forward. Listen and feel while the joints are in function.

Warning signs: TMJ dysfunction; movements should be smooth, continuous, and sound-free; both sides should function similarly and be free of pain.

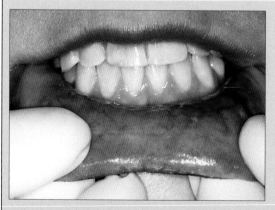

Anatomic location: Lips.

Method: Evert the lower lip so the gingival and mucobuccal fold is clearly visible. Dry gently with gauze. Inspect the inside of the lip. Palpate with thumb and index finger systematically from one corner of the mouth to the other. Repeat for the upper lip.

Warning signs: Changes in color, form, or texture of lips, vermillion border, and mucosal surfaces.

*Palpation of these areas can help detect suspicious changes and yield important medical information; however, these findings are less directly related to the oral cavity and perioral areas than other parts of the oral cancer examination. Palpation of these areas is a natural extension of the examination and is recommended.

Fig 3-3 Sequence of examination procedures (continued).

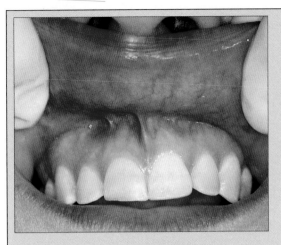

Anatomic location: Labial and alveolar mucosa, gingiva.

Method: Invert the labial tissue, dry with gauze, and inspect the mucosa. Inspect the gingival and alveolar mucosa. Palpate the labial mucosa using bilateral and bidigital compression; palpate the alveolar and gingival mucosa using digital compression.

Warning signs: Traumatic lesions, abrasions, signs of smokeless tobacco use, mucocele, vesiculoerosive disease, RAU, lesions.

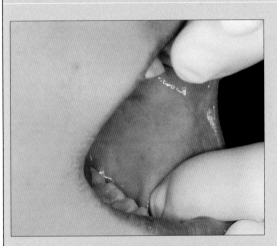

Anatomic location: Buccal mucosa.

Method: Have the patient turn the head to one side. Retract the cheek with fingers of one hand. Reflect light to inspect the mucosa from the commissure to retromolar area. Use a mouth mirror or tongue blade to visualize posterior areas. Palpate with thumb and first fingers bimanually. Repeat for the other side.

Warning signs: Traumatic lesions, cheek biting, lichen planus, leukoedema.

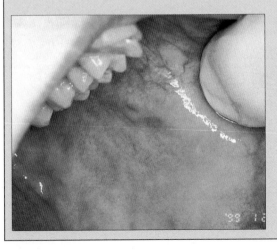

Anatomic location: Parotid gland.

Method: Palpate the gland and nodes bilaterally. Gently dry the opening of Stenson's duct with gauze; milk the gland by external compression. Observe salivary flow.

Warning signs: Gland dysfunction, sialolithiasis, parotitis, enlargements, tenderness, gland easily milked to express saliva.

Fig 3-3 Sequence of examination procedures (continued).

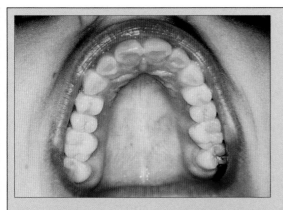

Anatomic location: Hard and soft palate, alveolar ridges.

Method: Have the patient tilt the head back slightly. Use a light source to visualize the area. Use a mirror or tongue blade to depress the tongue.

Warning signs: Hemorrhagic areas, discolorations, petechiae, denture and/or nicotine stomatitis, abscesses, fistulas, swellings.

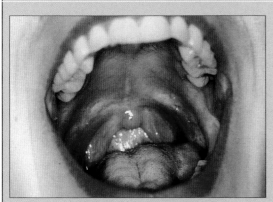

Anatomic location: Oropharynx (palatine and pharyngeal tonsils, posterior pharyngeal wall, uvula, anterior and posterior pillars).

Method: Have the patient relax the tongue; push on middle third of the tongue with a mirror or tongue blade; have the patient say "ah" and visually assess the area.

Warning signs: Signs of infection or disease, redness, swelling.

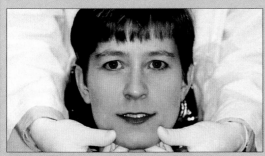

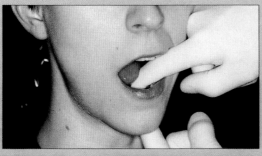

Anatomic location: Submental and submandibular glands (submental: in midline, behind tip of mandible).

Method: Tip the patient's head slightly down and forward to relax the tissues. "Cup" the mandible with thumb and fingers and palpate bilaterally. Draw tissue against the lateral border of the mandible. Use bidigital and circular compressions. Palpate from symphysis to the posterior border of the mandible.

Warning signs: Asymmetrical, irregular border of mandible; enlarged nodes, tenderness.

Fig 3-3 Sequence of examination procedures (continued).

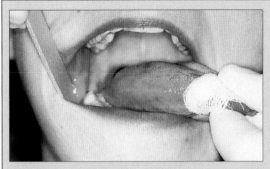

Anatomic location: Tongue (and lingual tonsils).[†]

Method: Inspect the dorsum while the tongue is at rest. Ask the patient to extend the tongue and move it from side to side. Firmly grasp the tongue with gauze and extend it for inspection while retracting the opposite cheek. Palpate along the exposed tongue surface. Palpate the lateral borders and lingual tonsils. Repeat for the opposite side. Have the patient touch the palate with the tip of the tongue to assess the ventral surface.

Warning signs: Papilla changes, asymmetry, vascularity, leukoplakia, nodal enlargements, erythroplakia.

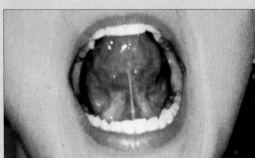

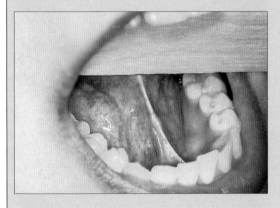

Anatomic location: Floor of the mouth.[†]

Method: Have the patient touch the palate with the tip of the tongue. Dry tissues with gauze. Palpate bimanually with one finger intraorally against the other hand under the chin. Test functioning of the submandibular gland by first drying Wharton's duct with gauze and externally compressing the gland to observe salivary flow.

Warning signs: Enlargement or masses, salivary gland blockage; asymmetry; tenderness, color changes, ankyloglossia.

Technique hints: (1) To view the tongue, a firmer grasp can be obtained by refolding a square piece of 2 x 2- or 4 x 4-inch gauze into a rectangular 1 x 6 or 2 x 12 strip. (2) Tongue blades and mouth mirrors are useful to visualize posterior regions of the mouth. Prior to their use, observe tissue where instruments will be placed, since these areas are frequently hidden from view. (3) Dry tissues present lesions more clearly. Because the appearance of lesions may be altered by saliva, gently dry the mucosal surface prior to examination. When dry, lesions appear more granular or slightly abraded. (4) Obstruction of Wharton's duct may cause enlargement of the submaxillary gland, which can mimic nodal involvement.

[†]To examine these areas, grasp the tongue with gauze and extend and distract it to one side to view exposed areas. For optimal viewing, apply external pressure on the submandibular gland on the same side.

Fig 3-3 Sequence of examination procedures (continued).

Identification of findings

Changes in tissue color, symmetry, texture, size, and contour need to be viewed with a high degree of suspicion and thoroughly evaluated to rule out malignancy. Any change detected must be described in detail, providing exact location, size, color, texture, and other significant characteristics. Suspicious areas should be palpated to assess the extent of invasiveness.[46] When possible, documentation with photographs is useful for follow-up comparisons.

When a lesion is detected, probable sources of irritation should be removed and, when present, the patient's use of alcohol and tobacco should be curtailed. Ten days to 2 weeks following the initial assessment, the patient needs to be reevaluated. Inflammatory lesions resulting from trauma or chronic irritation usually resolve or markedly improve within that time. Until proven otherwise, any lesion that persists with no apparent etiology should be considered suspicious.

When a lesion persists longer than 10 to 14 days, a diagnostic workup needs to be completed. This workup includes, but is not limited to, the use of diagnostic aids such as toluidine blue staining, cytology brushes, biopsy, and/or referral to an oral surgeon or oncologist (chapter 4). In addition, the patient needs to be made aware of the practitioner's concern and the need for immediate care. Finally, the diagnosis of oral cancer cannot be made without a definitive biopsy.

Summary

The stage at which oral cancer is diagnosed has a considerable impact on the patient's health and well-being. For those diagnosed with a lesion in an early stage, the associated morbidity and mortality is far less than for those with advanced lesions. To date, dentists and other health care providers have not offered comprehensive oral cancer examinations on a routine basis. Practice is determined largely by education. Continuing education courses are needed to provide clinicians with the information and practical applications to detect, diagnose, and manage oral cancer. Studies have documented that professionals with experience in detecting oral malignancies were more likely to identify a suspicious lesion than those with less experience.[56] The opportunities for oral cancer control are dramatically enhanced when a lesion is detected in an early stage.

On an annual basis, all patients need to undergo a comprehensive head and neck examination, including an assessment of their oral soft tissues. The recognition of early stage oral lesions requires constant awareness of the clinician as well as the patient. With ongoing continuing education programs, clinicians will be better able to detect subtle clinical changes, and with increased awareness, the public will be better informed and able to seek appropriate care.

Acknowledgment

Acknowledgment to Ms Jill A. Reynolds and Dr Mark W. Reynolds for modeling for the photographs in this manuscript.

References

1. Barasch A, Eisenberg E, Huang YW. Benign or malignant? A guide to the differential diagnosis of cancerous and non-cancerous oral lesions in older adults. Focus Adult Oral Health 1994;1:4.

2. Shugars DC, Patton LL. Detecting, diagnosing, and preventing oral cancer. Nurse Pract 1997;22:6.

3. Greene GW Jr. Detection and diagnosis of oral cancer. In: Carl W, Sako K (eds). Cancer and the Oral Cavity. Chicago: Quintessence, 1986:57–68.

4. Smart CR. Screening for cancer of the aerodigestive tract. Cancer 1993;72:3

5. Mashberg A, Samit A. Early diagnosis of asymptomatic oral and oropharyngeal squamous cancers. CA Cancer J Clin 1995;45:6.

6. Moore C. Anatomic origins and locations of oral cancer. Am J Surg 1967;114:510–513.

7. Mashberg A, Myers H. Anatomical site and size of 222 early asymptomatic oral squamous cell carcinomas. A continuing prospective study of oral cancer. Cancer 1976;37;2149–2157.

8. Marshall JR, Graham S, Haughey BP, Shedd D, O'Shea R, Brasure J, et al. Smoking, alcohol, dentition and diet in the epidemiology of oral cancer. Eur J Cancer B Oral Oncol 1992;28B;9.

9. Jones AS, Morar P, Phillips DE, Field JK, Husband D, Helliwell D, Helliwell TR. Second primary tumors in patients with head and neck squamous cell carcinoma. Cancer 1995;75:1343–1353.

10. McLaughlin JK, Gridley G, Block G, Winn DM, Preston-Martin S, Schoenberg JB, et al. Dietary factors in oral and pharyngeal cancer. J Natl Cancer Inst 1988;80;1237–1243.

11. Reynolds MW, Waheeb N, Yellowitz JA, Ord R. A typical (atypical) oral cancer. Presented at the Dental School Table Clinic, University of Maryland, April 22, 1998.

12. Silverman S. Oral Cancer, ed 4. American Cancer Society. Hamilton, Ontario: Decker, 1998.

13. Chen J, Eisenberg E, Krutchkoff DJ, Katz RV. Changing trends in oral cancer in the United States, 1935–1985: A Connecticut study. J Oral Maxillofac Surg 1991;49: 1152–1158.

14. Mashberg A, Barsa P. Screening for oral and oropharyngeal squamous carcinomas. Cancer 1984;34:5.

15. Maguire BT, Roberts EE. Dentists' examination of the oral mucosa to detect oral cancer [abstract]. J Public Health Dent 1994;54:115.

16. Pogrel MA. The dentist and oral cancer in the northeast of Scotland. Br Dent J 1974;137:15–20.

17. Coffin F. Cancer and the dental surgeon. Br Dent J 1964;161:199–202.

18. Mashberg A, Samit A. Early detection, diagnosis and management of oral and oropharyngeal cancer. Cancer 1989;39:67–88.

19. Prout MN, Morris SJ, Witzburg RA, Hurley C, Chatterjee S. A multidisciplinary educational program to promote head and neck cancer screening. J Cancer Educ 1992;7:2.

20. Yellowitz JA, Goodman HS. Assessing physicians' and dentists' oral cancer knowledge, opinions and practices. J Am Dent Assoc 1995;126:53–60.

21. Meskin LH. Oral cancer: The forgotten disease. J Am Dent Assoc 1994;125:1042–1045.

22. Epstein JB, Scully C. Assessing the patient at risk for oral squamous cell carcinoma. Spec Care Dentist 1997;17:4.

23. Centers for Disease Control and Prevention. Preventing and controlling oral and pharyngeal cancer. Recommendations from a national strategic planning conference. MMWR 1998;47(no. RR-14):1–12.

24. Gloeckler Ries LA, Kosary CL, Hankey BF, Miller BA, Harras A, Edwards BK (eds). SEER cancer statistics review, 1973–1994. Bethesda, MD: US Department of Health and Human Services, Public Health Service, National Institutes of Health, 1997. NIH pub no. 97-1789.

25. Spreight PM, Morgan PR. The natural history and pathology of oral cancer and precancer. Community Dent Health 1993;10(suppl 1):31–41.

26. Pommerenke FA, Weed DL. Physician compliance: Improving skills in preventive medicine practices. Am Fam Physician 1991;43:2.

27. Schnetler JF. Oral cancer diagnosis and delays in referral. Br J Oral Maxillofac Surg 1992;30:210–213.

28. Shafer WG. Initial mismanagement and delay in diagnosis of oral cancer. J Am Dent Assoc 1975;90: 1262–1264.

29. Sadowsky D, Kunzel C, Phelan J. Dentists' knowledge, case-finding behavior, and confirmed diagnosis of oral cancer. J Cancer Educ 1988;3:127–134.

30. Guggenheimer J, Verbin RS, Johnson JT, Horkowitz CA, Myers EN. Factors delaying the diagnosis of oral and oropharyngeal carcinomas. Cancer 1989;64: 932–935.

31. Yellowitz JA, Horowitz AM, Goodman HS, Canto MT, Farooq NS. Knowledge, opinions and practices of general dentists regarding oral cancer: A pilot survey. J Am Dent Assoc 1998;129:5.

32. Guggenheimer J, Hoffman RD. The importance of screening edentulous patients for oral cancer. J Prosthet Dent 1994;7:2.

33. Wildt J, Bundgaard T, Bentzen SM. Delay in the diagnosis of oral squamous cell carcinoma. Clin Otolaryngol 1995;20:21–25.

34. Scully C, Ward-Booth R. Detection and treatment of early cancers of the oral cavity. Crit Rev Oncol Hematol 1995;21:63–75.

35. Elwood JM, Gallagher RP. Factors influencing early diagnosis of cancer of the oral cavity. Can Med Assoc J 1985;133:651–656.

36. Prout MN, Barber CE, Morris SG, Geller AC, Koh HK. Use of health services before diagnosis of head and neck cancer among Boston residents. Am J Prev Med 1990;6:2.

37. Amsel Z, Engstrom PF, Strawitz JG. The dentist as a referral source of first episode head and neck cancer patients. J Am Dent Assoc 1983;106:195–197.

38. Love RR. The physician's role in cancer prevention and screening. Cancer Bull 1998;40:380–383.

39. Crissman JF, Gluckman J, Whiteley J, Quenell D. Squamous cell carcinoma of the floor of the mouth. Head Neck Surg 1980;3:2–7.

40. Lynch GR, Prout MN. Screening for cancer by residents in an internal medicine program. J Med Educ 1986;61:387–393.

41. Dimitroulis G, Reade P, Wiesenfeld D. Referral patterns of patients with oral squamous cell carcinoma, Australia. Eur J Cancer B Oral Oncol 1992;28B(1): 23–27.

42. Jovanovic A, Kostense PJ, Schulten EA, Snow GB, van der Waal I. Delay in diagnosis of oral squamous cell carcinoma: A report from The Netherlands. Eur J Cancer B Oral Oncol 992;28B(1):37–38.

43. Horowitz AM, Nourjah P, Gift HC. US adults' knowledge of risk factors and signs of oral cancers: 1990. J Am Dent Assoc 1995;126:39–45.

44. Coster JR, Foote RL, Olsen KD, Jack SM, Schaid DJ, DeSanto LW. Cervical nodal metastasis of squamous cell carcinoma of unknown origin: Indications for withholding radiation therapy. Int J Radiat Oncol Biol Phys 1992;23:743–749.

45. Marder MZ. The standard for care for oral diagnosis as it relates to oral cancer. Compendium 1998;19:6.

46. Shah JP, Lydiatt W. Treatment of cancer of the head and neck. CA Cancer J Clin 1995;45;352–368.

47. Darby ML, Walsh MM (eds). Dental Hygiene Theory and Practice. Philadelphia: Saunders, 1995.

48. Blot WJ, McLaughlin JK, Winn DM, et al. Smoking and drinking in relation to oral and pharyngeal cancer. Cancer Res 1988;48:3282–3287.

49. Gurenlian JR, Mc Fall DB, Mounts C, Williams C. Documenting oral cancer risk factors on health history forms [abstract]. J Dent Res 1966;75:306.

50. Yellowitz JA, Goodman HS, Horowitz AM, Al-Tannir MA. Assessment of alcohol and tobacco use in dental schools health history forms. J Am Dent Assoc 1995;59:1.

51. Goodman HS, Yellowitz JA, Horowitz AM. Oral cancer prevention: The role of family practitioners. Arch Fam Med 1995;4:628.

52. Alvi A. Oral cancer: How to recognize the danger signs. Postgrad Med 1996;99:4.

53. Bates B, Bickley LS, Hoekelman RA (eds). A Guide to Physical Examination and History Taking, ed 6. Philadelphia: JB Lippincott, 1995.

54. Shah JP. Patterns of cervical lymph node metastasis from squamous carcinomas of the upper aerodigestive tract. Am J Surg 1990;160:405–409.

55. Sonis ST, Fazio RC, Fang L (eds). Principles and Practice of Oral Medicine. Philadelphia: Saunders, 1995.

56. Julilen JA, Downer MC, Speight PM, Zakrzewska JM. Evaluation of health care workers' accuracy in recognising oral cancer and pre-cancer. Int Dent J 1996; 46:4.

CHAPTER 4

Diagnostic Procedures

Robert A. Ord, DDS, MD, MS

Diagnostic procedures are used when indicated following a carefully taken history and examination of the head and neck (see chapter 3). Any patient with an ulcer, a mass, or any other undiagnosed lesion present for 3 weeks or more should be suspected of having cancer, especially if the patient is in a high-risk group (eg, elderly, tobacco user, and/or alcohol consumer). In many cases the diagnosis will be obvious, with a large granular ulcer with rolled edges and associated hard cervical nodes. However, early cancers may be subtle red or white lesions that may initially be treated as inflammatory or infectious. Delay in diagnosis will adversely affect the prognosis; therefore, the clinician must be highly suspicious of lesions that do not respond to conservative therapy. Diagnostic procedures include noninvasive radiologic studies and biopsy.

Radiologic Studies in the Patient with Oral Cancer

When the suspected cancer involves the jaws, radiographs, such as panoral or periapical views, may provide valuable information. Although early cortical invasion is not clearly visible on radiographs,[1] more extensive involvement is seen as a diffuse bone lysis with a moth-eaten irregular appearance (Figs 4-1a and 4-1b). The teeth are relatively resistant to this destruction. There is a great deal of controversy regarding which imaging technique is best for the accurate diagnosis of early bone invasion.[2] It is generally agreed that computed tomography (CT) can depict cortical invasion better than magnetic resonance imaging (MRI), which provides the best image of bone marrow spread.[3,4]

When the jaws are affected by sarcomas (eg, osteosarcoma), a periapical radiograph that shows widening of the periodontal membrane may be the earliest diagnostic sign (Fig 4-2).[5] These tumors cause diffuse bone destruction, with lytic and occasionally sclerotic areas. In Ewing's sarcoma, subperiosteal bone may be deposited to give an onionskin appearance. Although metastases to the jaws are rare, cancer of the breast, lung, kidney, prostate, and thyroid often involve the facial bones, particularly the mandible. Although moth-eaten rarefaction is a classic finding, occasionally lesions may be "punched out" in appearance (Fig 4-3). Such a lesion, accompanied by numbness of the lower lip, is always a sinister sign. Prostatic metastases are unusual in that they often show sclerotic areas.

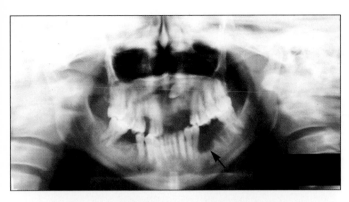

Fig 4-1a Early erosive lesion on the crest of the ridge in the left mandibular premolar region *(arrow).*

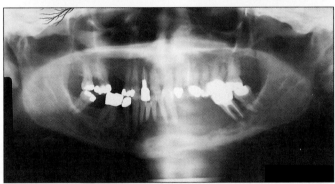

Fig 4-1b Extensive bony destruction and loss of teeth due to oral carcinoma.

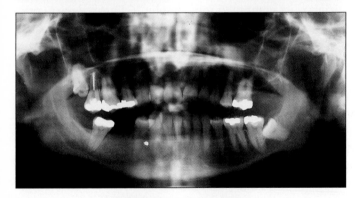

Fig 4-2 Widened periodontal ligament on the mandibular right second molar. Also note the irregular inferior alveolar canal.

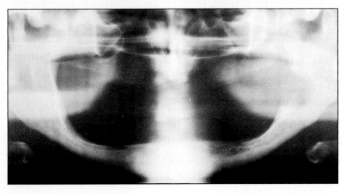

Fig 4-3 Metastatic lesion from breast cancer. The patient presented with numbness of the left lower lip.

Fig 4-4a Extensive tumor in the left maxilla.

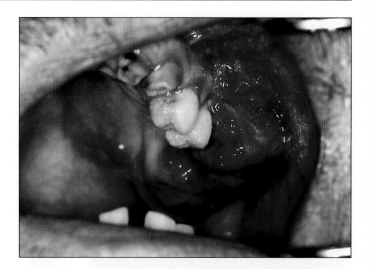

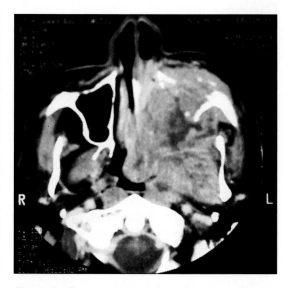

Fig 4-4b Computed tomographic scan showing tumor involvement of the maxillary sinus and nasal cavity and destruction of the posterior bony maxilla with involvement of the pterygoids.

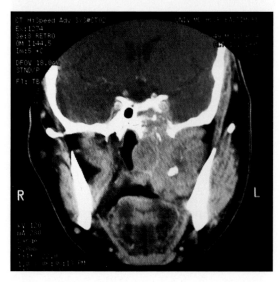

Fig 4-4c Coronal CT scan showing invasion of the skull base, involving the sphenoid and cavernous sinus.

Lesions involving the maxilla are always best depicted using CT or MRI because the extent of involvement of the paranasal sinuses, orbit, and skull base is usually not evident on clinical examination or radiographs (Figs 4-4a to 4-4c). The ability to assess invasion of the pterygoid musculature and skull base fre-quently determines the feasibility of surgery. Magnetic resonance images are more useful in differentiating tumor involvement from mucus in the obstructed sinus.

Other imaging modalities that have been used to assess early bone involvement by can-cer include the isotope bone scan. This

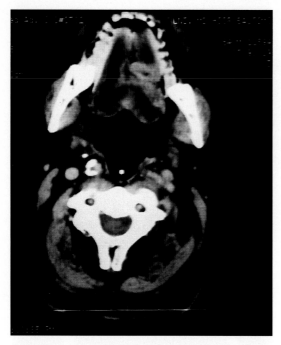

Fig 4-5 CT scan showing carcinoma of the tongue, extending deeply and crossing the midline.

method yields a high incidence of false-positive results, but when it is negative it rules out invasion. Although the soft tissues are not well depicted by radiographs, other imaging techniques give valuable information regarding both the primary tumor and cervical nodal metastases. Both CT and MRI have been used to assess muscle invasion, especially in the tongue (Fig 4-5).[6] Both modalities are widely used to help diagnose lymph node involvement because clinical examination of the neck is only 70% accurate. The use of these techniques has increased diagnostic accuracy to greater than 90%.

The CT criteria for nodal metastasis are nodes in the submandibular triangle or jugulodigastric region with a diameter greater than 1.5 cm, or any other cervical node with a diameter greater that 1 cm; nodes that are

rounded or spherical; or nodes with central necrosis.[7] These scans are particularly useful for obese patients or those undergoing radiation therapy. However, neither CT nor MRI has the ability to depict microscopic disease, and a negative scan result cannot rule out occult cancer in the neck.

Another imaging technique that has been used in the head and neck is ultrasound. This modality has been used to assess the thickness of primary tumors and to depict metastatic lymph nodes.

Biopsy

Histologic confirmation of the diagnosis of cancer is an absolute requirement prior to commencing any treatment with surgery, radiation therapy, or chemotherapy. As previously mentioned, any oral lesion present for 3 weeks or more with an unknown diagnosis requires biopsy to confirm or refute the presence of a malignancy. In a large lesion, incisional biopsy with local anesthesia and use of a scalpel or scissors is the standard procedure. When the lesion is vascular, or if the surgeon prefers, a carbon-dioxide laser may be used for the biopsy to reduce bleeding. However, the pathologist should be informed that a laser was used, because this can cause artifacts that may confuse the diagnosis. Although obtaining a pie-shaped biopsy specimen at the tumor edge, providing a sample of normal mucosa as well as tumor, is classically taught, the diagnosis can be made from a biopsy specimen within the lesion that does not include surrounding normal tissue. Obviously if there is central ulceration and necrosis, a biopsy specimen of this area will fail to provide representative tissue, and a nondiagnostic histologic study will result.

Fast-growing lesions are often friable and vascular, and in these cases sutures tend to cut through the tumor tissue. Biopsies of these tumors are often impossible to close primarily and can cause troublesome bleeding. In such cases, it is preferable to include normal mucosa, which can be sutured, in the biopsy margins. In exophytic or verrucous lesions, the biopsy must be deep enough to include submucosa to show invasion. Indeed, verrucous carcinoma is cytologically benign, and failure to obtain a deep enough specimen that shows the advancing invasive front may lead to an incorrect diagnosis. When a tumor shows extensive submucosal spread, the excision must extend deep enough through the normal tissue to make sure the cancerous tissue is sampled.

Biopsy data and dilemmas

Even with a well-taken biopsy specimen, it is important to ensure that sufficient information is given to the pathologist to help with diagnosis. Data such as age, site, appearance, smoking habits, history of the lesion, and the clinician's provisional diagnosis will aid the pathologist and become invaluable in a difficult case.[8] The clinician has the opportunity to observe and monitor the lesion. If the initial histologic diagnosis is benign, but the lesion continues to grow and behave like a malignancy, further biopsies at a different site should be performed. It is a mistake to accept one benign biopsy result if this does not correspond to the lesion's biologic behavior. Even in experienced hands, sampling error may mean that two or three repeat biopsy procedures are necessary to obtain the correct diagnosis.

Another dilemma faced by clinicians is when a widespread lesion has different appearances throughout, including red, white, and granular areas. In this type of lesion it may be difficult to discern which areas are dysplastic and which represent invasive squa-

mous cell carcinoma. It is helpful to perform multiple "geographic biopsies" at different sites to clearly define the pathologic changes. Geographic biopsies are helpful in tumors with ill-defined margins where sampling different sites may define the extent of the tumor. A different method of dealing with this problem is the use of toluidine blue (vide infra). However, a large lesion provides fewer biopsy problems than a small lesion.

When lesions are 1 cm or less, the clinician may be tempted to excise the entire lesion, rather than perform an incisional biopsy. The former practice provides no more information than a properly performed incisional biopsy and may lead to increased morbidity (and even mortality) for the patient. It is clear that margins of less than 5 mm around the cancerous tissue are associated with increased recurrence rates and should be regarded as positive cancerous margins.[9-11] Therefore, an excisional margin of 1 cm is recommended at most oral sites for squamous cell carcinoma, although 1.5- to 2-cm margins may be necessary for squamous cell carcinoma of the tongue.[12,13] This means that a 1 × 1-cm lesion requires an excisional biopsy measuring 3 × 3 cm and 1 cm deep to the deepest area of the neoplasm, for cure. When excisional biopsy is undertaken in this fashion for small lesions, good results are obtained.[14]

In the common scenario, when excisional biopsy is undertaken with only a few millimeters of margin, all margins are positive for cancer; subsequent closure distorts the tissues and may push cancer cells deeper. If the patient is then referred to another surgeon for definitive treatment or is not seen for a few weeks, the biopsy site will have healed, leaving the surgeon no obvious tumor or margin to excise. The subsequent surgical excision usually consists of a large block of tissue in the area, as the surgeon attempts to "guess" where the cancer was and to remove the microscop-

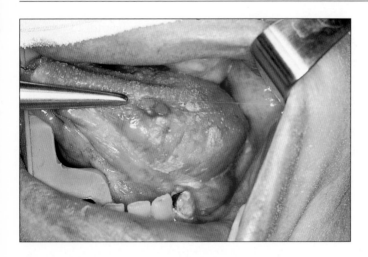

Fig 4-6a Extensive leukoplakia of the tongue and floor of the mouth in an elderly woman. Pointer shows site of previous tongue biopsy with early focus of carcinoma.

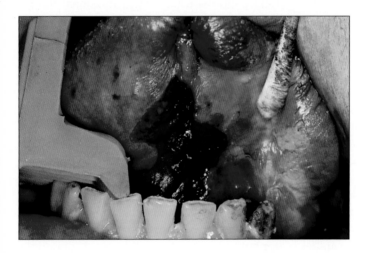

Fig 4-6b Toluidine blue rinse showing a deeply staining lesion on the floor of the mouth, which was an infiltrating squamous cell carcinoma separate from the tongue cancer.

ic residual disease. Thus the excisional biopsy is harmful rather than helpful and should not be undertaken where cancer is suspected.

Identification of biopsy site

A useful adjunct to help the clinician decide which suspicious areas of the oral mucosa require biopsy is the use of the vital stain toluidine blue. This stain may be used as a rinse to screen the entire oral cavity, or may be topically applied to areas of concern. Invasive carcinoma and carcinoma in situ stain dark blue, but dysplasia stains variably. This technique is especially useful in patients with widespread panleukoplakia or erythroplakia (Figs 4-6a to 4-6d), or in patients who have received previous radiation therapy or surgery and are at risk from recurrence but are difficult to evaluate clinically. The stain may be used to visualize lesions in the faucial or tonsillar region that

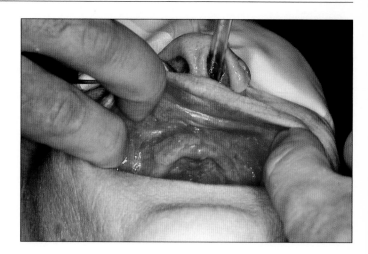

Fig 4-6c Carcinoma of the cheek and an indistinct red and white lesion on the anterior alveolar ridge and palate in an 80-year-old woman.

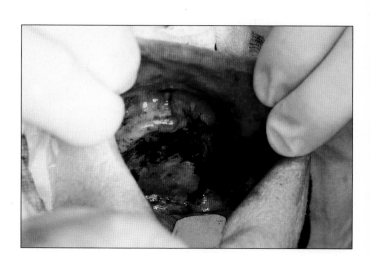

Fig 4-6d Toluidine blue rinse delineating the extent of carcinoma in situ, dysplasia, and early carcinoma.

may be difficult to examine. Toluidine blue has also been used to define the margins of cancer.[15]

Mashberg[16] compared topical toluidine application to the rinse and found the topical application superior, with 5.7% false-positive results and 2.5% false-negative results, compared to 9.2% false-positive results and 11.1% false-negative results for the toluidine rinse. Best results are obtained by the use of a 1% acetic acid rinse to reduce retention of the dye by the dorsum of the tongue, plaque, exfoliated keratin, or traumatic ulceration. Restaining 14 days after the initial test to allow inflammation to resolve in equivocal cases reduces false-positive results. The classic reported technique[17] involves two 20-second oral rinses, followed by a 20-second rinse with 1% acetic acid. The mucosa is dried with gauze and 1% toluidine blue is applied topically (or rinsed) for 1 to 2 minutes. A final 1-minute rinse with 1% acetic acid completes the sequence. In combining six

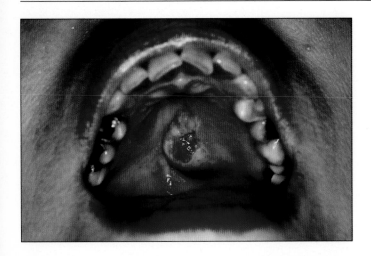

Fig 4-7 Minor salivary tumor of the palate shows central ulceration from biopsy.

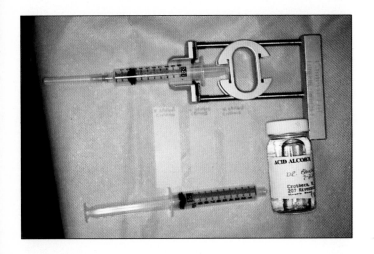

Fig 4-8a Instrumentation for fine needle aspiration biopsy. Note the syringe holder.

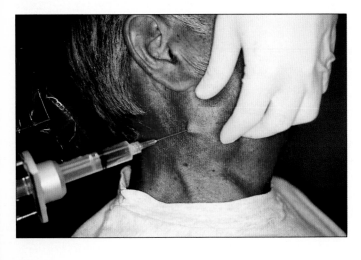

Fig 4-8b Aspiration with a syringe holder, which allows the mass to be stabilized with one hand while aspirating with the other hand.

separate studies comprising 1,071 patients, a sensitivity of 96% to 100% and a specificity of 87% to 100% was reported.[18]

Biopsy technique modification

When other types of cancer occur, biopsy techniques require modification. Salivary gland tumors present as submucosal masses mostly involving the junction of the hard and soft palate. In these tumors, biopsy should be performed in the center of the lesion so the margins are not compromised, because the overlying mucosa will be excised when the tumor is resected (Fig 4-7).[19] When the clinician suspects a lymphoma (eg, a soft irregular tumor at the junction of the hard and soft palate) or an usual tumor in a patient with HIV, part of the biopsy specimen should be sent fresh or in saline (not frozen or in formalin) to allow for cytogenetic studies and typing.

Fine needle aspiration biopsy is a quick, inexpensive, accurate, and easily performed technique that can help diagnose metastases in enlarged cervical nodes in the patient with oral cancer.[20] A 10-mL syringe, a 22-gauge needle, a syringe holder that allows aspiration with one hand, microscope slides, and a bottle of 95% alcohol fixative are all that is required. The barrel of the syringe is drawn back 1 to 2 mL, and the skin overlying the mass is prepared with iodine. The needle is inserted into the neck mass, which is stabilized with one hand, while the other hand applies suction to the syringe in its holder. The needle is moved up and down through the mass, fragmenting cells and maintaining suction. (The needle is not withdrawn from the mass; Figs 4-8a and 4-8b.) Suction is released and the needle withdrawn. One drop of fluid is expressed onto the microscope slide (preferably a frosted glass slide), smeared

using another slide, and placed in the alcohol fixative. If there is sufficient material, two to three slides can be prepared. It should be remembered that a negative result does not mean there is no cancer, but a positive result is diagnostic.

In a comprehensive review of the literature on head and neck fine needle aspiration, Abaza and Miloro[21] found the sensitivity and specificity rates for a malignant diagnosis to be over 90%.

Summary

The imaging and biopsy techniques described in this chapter are important in the diagnosis and staging of oral cancer. In addition, as part of the workup, chest radiographs and liver function tests are used as screens for distant metastases. Routine blood tests and electro-cardiography to determine fitness for anesthesia and other tests as indicated by the medical history are also performed. Usually, endoscopic examination of the larynx, pharynx, lungs, and esophagus of patients with oral cancer is carried out. These patients have a high incidence of second upper aerodigestive tract primary cancer because of their histories of tobacco and alcohol abuse. Following this testing, the cancer is staged and the most appropriate treatment plan discussed.

References

1. Brown J, Griffith P, Browne R. A comparison of different imaging modalities after periosteal stripping in predicting the invasion of the mandible by oral squamous cell carcinoma. Br J Oral Maxillofac Surg 1994; 32:347.

2. Ord RA, Samardi M, Papadimitrou J. A comparison of segmental and marginal bone resection for oral squamous cell carcinoma involving the mandible. J Oral Maxillofac Surg 1997;55:470–477.

3. Van Den Brekel MWM, Castelijns JA, Snow GB. The role of modern imaging studies in staging and therapy of head and neck neoplasms. Semin Oncol 1994;3: 340.

4. Castelijns JA, Van Den Brekel MWM. Magnetic resonance imaging evaluation of extracranial head and neck tumors. Magn Reson Q 1993;2:113.

5. Gardener DG, Mills DM. The widened periodontal ligament of osteosarcoma of the jaws. Oral Surg 1976;41:652–656.

6. Fruehwald FX. Clinical examination, C.T., US in tongue cancer staging. Eur J Radiol 1995;50: 533–540.

7. Som PM. Lymph nodes of the neck. Radiology 1987; 165:593.

8. Whitesides LM, Ferrierra LR, Ord RA. Audit of clinical information and diagnosis supplied to the pathologist following biopsy of oral squamous cell carcinomas. J MD State Dent Assoc 1995;38:63–65.

9. Looser KG, Shah JP, Strong EW. The significance of "positive" margins in surgically resected epidermoid carcinomas. Head Neck 1978;1:107.

10. Chen TY, Emrich LJ, Driscoll DL. The clinical significance of pathological findings in surgically resected margins of the primary tumor in the head and neck carcinomas. Int J Radiat Oncol Biol Phys 1987;13:833.

11. Ord RA, Aisner S. Accuracy of frozen sections in assessing margins in oral cancer resection. J Oral Maxillofac Surg 1997;55:663–669.

12. Harrisson, DFN. The questionable value of total glossectomy. Head Neck Surg 1983;6:632.

13. Yeun PW, Lam KY, Chan ACL, Wei WI, Lam LK. Clinicopathologic analysis of local spread of carcinoma of the tongue. Am J Surg 1998;175:242–244.

14. Stell PM, Wood GD, Scott MH. Early oral cancer: Treatment by biopsy excision. Br J Oral Surg 1982;20:234–238.

15. Portugal LC, Wilson KM, Biddinger PW, Gluckman JL. The role of the toluidine blue in assessing margin status after resection of squamous cell carcinomas of the upper aerodigestive tract. Arch Otolarnyngol Head Neck Surg 1996;122:517–519.

16. Mashberg A. Final evaluation of tolonium chloride rinse for screening of high-risk patients with asymptomatic squamous carcinoma. J Am Dent Assoc 1983; 106:319.

17. Mashberg A, Sanit A. Early detection, diagnosis, and management of oral and oropharyngeal cancer. CA Cancer J Clin 1989;39:67.

18. Clayman L. Management of mucosal premalignant lesions. Oral Maxillofac Clin North Am 1994;3: 431–444.

19. Ord RA. Management of intra-oral salivary gland tumors. Oral Maxillofac Surg Clin North Am 1994; 3:499–522.

20. Slack RUT, Croft CB, Croove LP. Fine needle aspiration cytology in the management of head and neck masses. Clin Otolaryngol 1985;10:93–96.

21. Abaza NA, Miloro M. Fine-needle aspiration in oral and maxillofacial diagnosis. Oral Maxillofac Surg Clin North Am 1994;3:401.

CHAPTER 5

Premalignant Lesions

Michael A. Siegel, DDS, MS

Leukoplakia

Leukoplakia is a clinical term that describes a white lesion on the oral mucosa that cannot be scraped off and cannot be classified as another clinically diagnosable disease. The majority of these lesions are detected in individuals in their 50s, 60s, and 70s, although patients of any age may be affected. About half of the lesions involve the mandibular mucosa, mandibular sulcus, and buccal mucosa.[1] The traditional male predisposition to such lesions is decreasing, and women are affected almost as frequently as men.

The majority of leukoplakias are physiologic reactions of the mucosa to chronic trauma or irritation. Ill-fitting dentures and parafunctional oral habits such as cheek or tongue chewing are common causes (Figs 5-1a and 5-1b). Leukoplakic lesions are also found in patients with a history of tobacco or alcohol use. Other factors associated with these white mucosal lesions include mechanical and chemical irritants, chronic candidiasis, syphilis, and electrogalvanic reactions.[2] The clinical appearance of leukoplakia varies. The lesions may appear smooth, fissured, or corrugated, and white, gray, or translucent. Leukoplakias also vary with regard to size and distribution. They may be barely discernible clinically or cover entire mucosal surfaces. The sites where leukoplakic lesions are commonly encountered are the floor of the mouth, lateral and ventral borders of the tongue, labial and buccal mucosas, gingivas, the soft palate, and the retromolar area.

The majority of leukoplakias (80%) are benign.[1] The remaining lesions are either premalignant (dysplastic or carcinoma in situ) (Fig 5-2) or malignant (Fig 5-3). Dysplastic lesions are multicentric and are most commonly encountered in the floor of the mouth or on the tongue.[1,3] Other risk sites for premalignant or malignant leukoplakias include the lip, lateral and ventral borders of the tongue, floor of the mouth, soft palate, uvula, and retromolar areas. Leukoplakic lesions are prognostically ominous in a patient with a history of carcinoma of the tongue. Multiple carcinomas of the oral cavity and oropharynx (116 times greater than expected) have been encountered in patients with a history of tongue carcinoma.[4] The clinician faces the

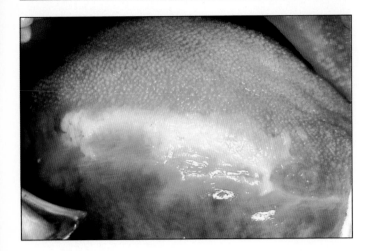

Fig 5-1a Linear leukoplakia of the right lateral tongue border in a patient with a tongue-biting habit.

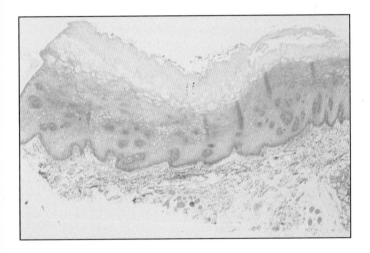

Fig 5-1b Hyperorthokeratosis, acanthosis, and mild chronic inflammation. (Hematoxylin and eosin stain. Original magnification ×35.)

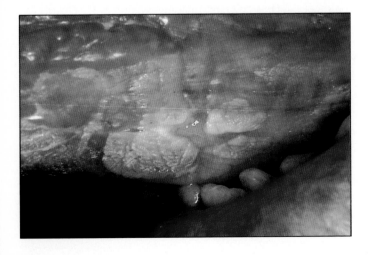

Fig 5-2a Leukoplakia of the left lateral tongue border.

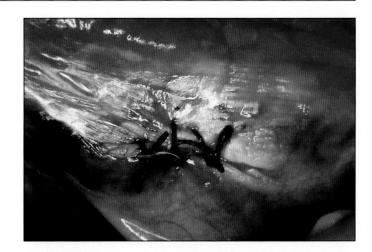

Fig 5-2b Suture placement following incisional biopsy.

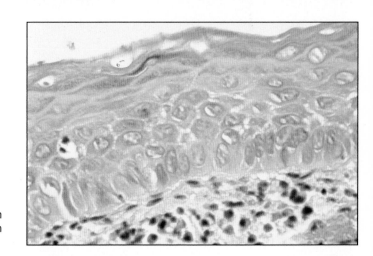

Fig 5-2c Mild dysplasia. (Hematoxylin and eosin stain. Original magnification ×100.)

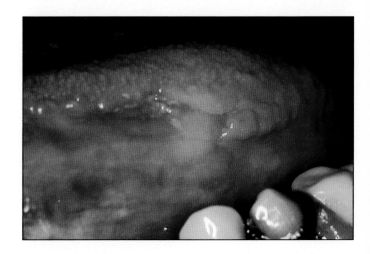

Fig 5-2d Appearance of tongue following 6 weeks of topical retinoid therapy.

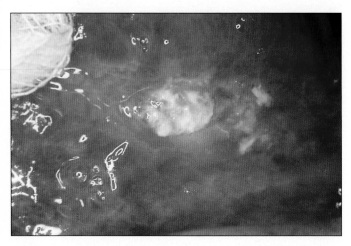

Fig 5-3a Leukoplakia of the left lateral tongue border similar in appearance to the lesion in Fig 5-2a.

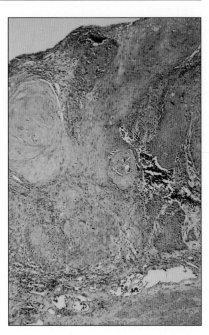

Fig 5-3b Well-differentiated squamous cell carcinoma. (Hematoxylin and eosin stain. Original magnification ×40.)

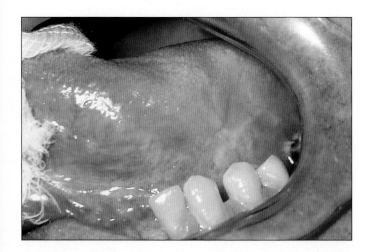

Fig 5-3c Appearance of tongue border 9 months after surgical resection.

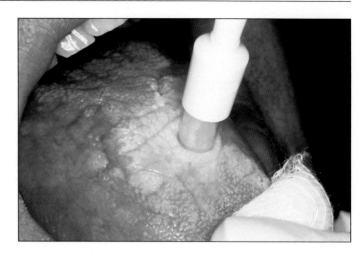

Fig 5-4 Punch biopsy instrument.

problem of determining which of these lesions are premalignant or malignant and must determine the nature of the white lesion without unreasonably alarming the patient.

The initial step in the treatment of leukoplakia is to eliminate any source of chronic irritation or trauma, such as a sharp tooth or denture border. Controversy exists as to whether a therapeutic trial of medication such as a topical steroid or retinoid is appropriate prior to biopsy.[5] If the leukoplakic lesion has not resolved within 2 to 4 weeks following the removal of local causative factors, biopsy should be performed to establish the diagnosis. The clinician should submit one or more tissue specimens excised from sites representing the clinical lesion for histopathologic evaluation. Accurate, reproducible agreement of microscopic diagnosis of oral epithelial dysplasia is difficult to achieve, even among experienced board-certified oral pathologists.[6] It is therefore essential that the clinician provide the pathologist with biopsy specimens accompanied by an accurate history of the lesion.

Biopsy can be performed using either a conventional scalpel or a punch technique. Punch biopsy instruments are reminiscent of round to ovoid cookie cutters. They are commercially available in a variety of diameters and are disposable after a single use. Punch biopsy instruments enable the clinician to remove a known size of tissue without a scalpel (Fig 5-4). Small lesions can be excised, whereas larger lesions should be incised. If lesions suspected of being malignant are completely excised, sutures must remain in place until a definitive histopathologic diagnosis is received. In cases of malignancy that necessitate further surgery to achieve appropriate tissue margins, the sutures serve as a marker of the biopsy site. Unfortunately, if the excisional biopsy is allowed to heal without sutures remaining in place, the surgeon will be unable to determine the site of the tumor. This necessitates a more radical surgical procedure to ensure that the entire tumor has been removed.

Erythroleukoplakia

Leukoplakia with localized red-speckled areas or erythroplakia with localized white-speckled areas also confers a high risk of oral cancer

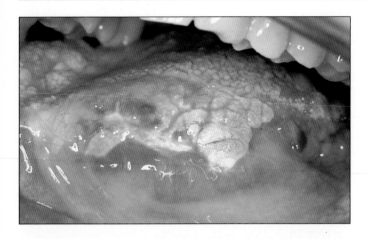

Fig 5-5a Erythroleukoplakia of the left lateral tongue border. Note the velvety red appearance admixed among the leukoplakic plaques.

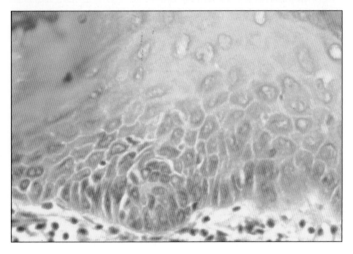

Fig 5-5b Moderate dysplasia. (Hematoxylin and eosin stain. Original magnification ×100.)

(Figs 5-5a and 5-5b). Many terms have been used to describe these red-and-white-mixed lesions, such as *speckled leukoplakia* or *speckled erythroplakia*. There is a fourfold increased risk that these lesions will undergo malignant transformation when compared to homogeneous leukoplakias.[7] Erythroleukoplakia may occur in any intraoral site and has a male predilection. These lesions are usually found in patients who use tobacco and alcohol and exhibit poor oral hygiene. *Candida albicans*, a commonly encountered intraoral fungal organism, is often found in these lesions and may have a role in the dysplastic changes.[7] However, no studies have documented a direct relationship between candidal involvement and malignant transformation.[2,8] Red-and-white-mixed lesions that have not resolved following removal of any local causative factors should be selected for biopsy due to their increased risk for developing into carcinoma.

Erythroplakia

Erythroplakia is a clinical term used to define a velvety red patch that cannot be characterized as any other condition. These lesions are often asymptomatic and are first recognized

Fig 5-6 Multifocal erythroplakia in a 73-year-old man. Biopsy revealed carcinoma in situ of the palate and well-differentiated squamous cell carcinoma of the tongue and labial commissure.

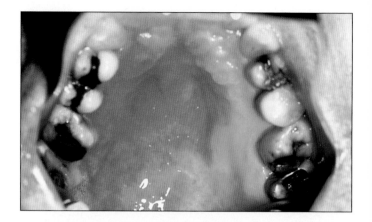

Fig 5-6a Palate.

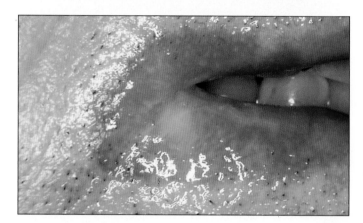

Fig 5-6b Labial commissure.

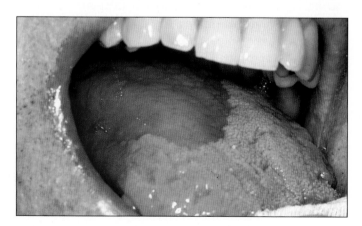

Fig 5-6c Tongue dorsum.

during a routine dental examination. Erythroplakias can occur anywhere in the oral cavity but are found most often in the floor of the mouth and oropharynx (Figs 5-6a to 5-6c). The redness is due to the thinning (erosion) of overlying epithelium. Men and women over the age of 60 may be equally affected.

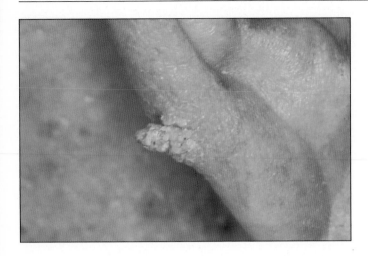

Fig 5-7 Actinic keratosis on the ear. Note the rough, keratotic surface texture.

Biopsy of erythroplakic lesions is mandatory, because it has been shown histologically that approximately 90% represent severe dysplasia, carcinoma in situ, or carcinoma.[9] The patient must be observed closely since multiple sites of the oral cavity may be affected, a phenomenon referred to as *field cancerization*. In patients with multiple lesions, representative biopsy specimens must be procured from each site.

Actinic Cheilitis

Actinic keratosis is a premalignant skin condition associated with cutaneous epithelial cells resulting from chronic exposure to sunlight (Fig 5-7). When it affects the lower lip, this condition is referred to as actinic (solar) cheilitis. Chronic exposure to sunlight is probably the causative factor for the wide geographic distribution of actinic cheilitis and the lip cancer that may result from this disorder.[10] It is characterized as atrophy, crusting, and/or

ulceration at the junction of the skin and vermilion zone of the lower lip (Fig 5-8). The clinical appearance of the lip is not a reliable indicator of premalignant or malignant changes within the lip.[11] Approximately 10% of actinic cheilitis undergoes malignant change; therefore, a biopsy must be performed if lesions do not resolve when sunlight exposure is reduced and sunscreens are used.[12] Management of actinic cheilitis consists of surgical excision, lip shave, or use of either topical retinoids or 5-fluorouracil.

Lichen Planus

Oral lichen planus (OLP) is a disorder of unknown etiology and represents the most common dermatologic disease with oral manifestations. The skin lesions present as violaceous papules with a fine scale occurring most commonly on the flexor surface of the arms and legs. The oral lesions vary greatly in

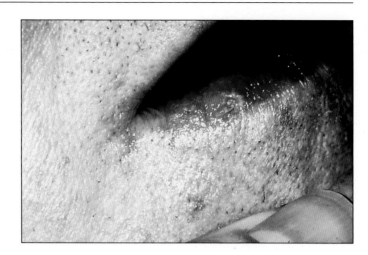

Fig 5-8 Actinic cheilitis. Note the ulceration and crusting of the vermilion zone.

appearance and frequently represent the only clinical sign of disease. Lichen planus is usually found in patients older than 40 years. The patient may be unaware of the intraoral form of the disease because it is often asymptomatic. Therefore, the oral soft tissues of patients with signs and symptoms of dermal lichen planus must be examined. The differential diagnosis of oral lichen planus should include discoid lupus and lichenoid drug reaction.[13,14]

Oral lichen planus may be seen in a variety of clinical forms. The majority of OLP lesions are identified by the presence of fine, reticular white lines (Wickham's striae) on the lateral borders of the tongue, buccal mucosa, and gingiva. However, striae are not always present, especially in the ulcerative form of the disease.

Atrophic lesions of the gingiva also may be noted in these patients, and on occasion, fluid-filled blisters (bullous type) may be encountered. Therefore, definitive diagnosis is made with a biopsy.

Reports have associated OLP with malignant transformation (Figs 5-9a to 5-9c). There is debate about whether OLP is a precancerous condition.[15,16] In three large prospective clinical studies of 570, 214, and 95 patients with OLP conducted by Silverman et al,[17–19] malignant transformation occurred in 1.2%, 2.3%, and 3.2%, respectively. It is suggested that a biopsy be taken of OLP lesions that persist following therapy and are red and/or ulcerated to ensure against malignant transformation. All patients with OLP should be reevaluated on a regular basis.

Smokeless Tobacco

Smokeless tobacco may be used in the form of either chewing tobacco or snuff. The resulting lesions appear as wrinkled, corrugated areas of the mandibular alveolar mucosa at the vestibular fornices (Fig 5-10a). These sites may take on a white to yellow coloration.

Fig 5-9 Lichen planus and well-differentiated squamous cell carcinoma in a 35-year-old man.

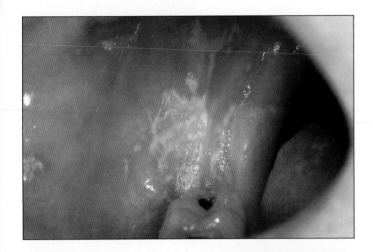

Fig 5-9a Reticular lichen planus of the right posterior buccal mucosa.

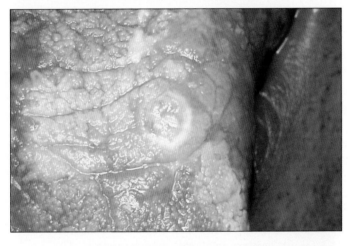

Fig 5-9b Painless, ulcerated papule on the left tongue dorsum.

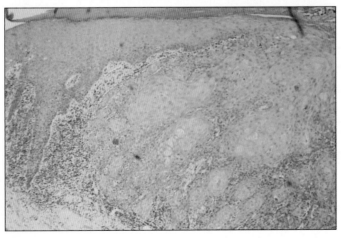

Fig 5-9c Photomicrograph revealing lichen planus on the left side of the field and well-differentiated squamous cell carcinoma on the right side. (Hematoxylin and eosin stain. Original magnification ×40.)

Fig 5-10 Smokeless tobacco–associated lesions.

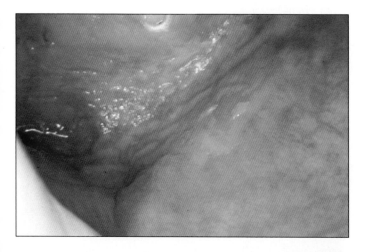

Fig 5-10a Corrugated appearance of the mucobuccal fold.

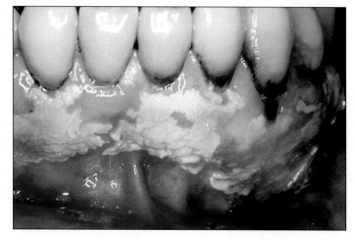

Fig 5-10b Leukoplakic plaque on the gingiva.

Frank leukoplakic lesions of the mandibular gingival tissues may also be encountered (Fig 5-10b). These lesions are consistent with the site of tobacco placement. A sixfold increased risk of leukoplakia was noted in smokeless tobacco users when compared to nonusers.[20]

These lesions have been associated with dysplasia, verrucous carcinoma, and epidermoid carcinoma.[21] Therefore, patients must be encouraged to discontinue the use of these products, and a biopsy of any unre-solved site should be performed within 1 month. Patients who continue to use smokeless tobacco must be reevaluated at regular intervals. Patients with mucosal lesions who are unwilling to discontinue the use of smokeless tobacco products should be instructed to place the tobacco in a different intraoral location for 2 to 4 weeks. This allows for resolution of the mucosal lesion. A biopsy of any unresolved lesions should be performed.

Fig 5-11 Proliferative verrucous leukoplakia in a 59-year-old woman.

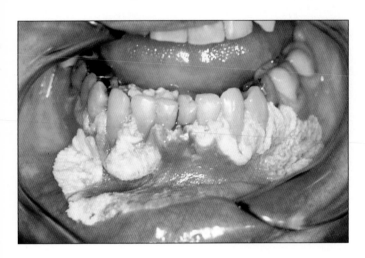

Fig 5-11a Overview of the mandibular arch. Note the bilateral distribution of the exophytic lesions.

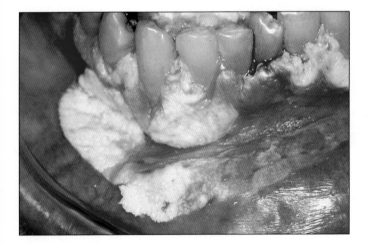

Fig 5-11b Close-up view of the right canine area.

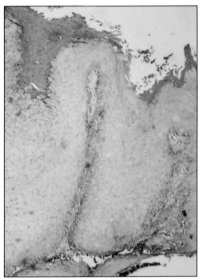

Fig 5-11c Photomicrograph disclosing verrucous carcinoma. (Hematoxylin and eosin stain. Original magnification ×40.)

Proliferative Verrucous Leukoplakia

Proliferative verrucous leukoplakia (PVL) is a clinical term for a group of lesions that tends to persist or expand and is associated with a high risk of malignant transformation.[22,23] They are recognized as being white, exophytic, fissured, and present in multiple intraoral sites (Figs 5-11a to 5-11c). Histopathologically, these lesions represent a clinical spectrum ranging from benign hyperorthokeratosis (callous) to verrucous carcinoma to invasive squamous cell carcinoma, and on this basis are graded on a scale from 1 to 10. While this is a heterogenous histologic spectrum, it appears that PVL is a very high-risk precancerous lesion with high transformation and mortality rates. Women are affected more frequently than men and tobacco use is associated with fewer than one third of these cases.

Early biopsy is mandatory for these lesions. Definitive treatment includes total surgical excision or laser ablation. Regular follow-up care is necessary.

Human Papillomavirus

Human papillomavirus (HPV) infections may occur intraorally as verruca vulgaris, condyloma acuminatum, and focal epithelial hyperplasia (Heck's disease). It is not known whether all intraoral squamous papillomas are etiologically related to cutaneous verruca vulgaris. However, some intraoral papillary lesions are associated with HPV. Presently over 70 specific forms of HPV have been identified. Types 16 and 18 are termed *oncoviruses* because they are associated with malignant transformation.[24] However, their role in the development of oral cancer is not clear.

Cutaneous verruca vulgaris (common warts) are found on the skin. Autoinoculation of the lips, tongue, gingiva, and palate may occur if the patient bites these lesions off the skin surface (Figs 5-12a to 5-12d). Oral squamous papillomas may be sessile or pedunculated and have a characteristic rough, pebbly surface. Surgical removal is the treatment of choice for intraoral lesions. This allows histopathologic examination of the specimen for viral epithelial changes. Skin lesions may be removed surgically, using liquid nitrogen, with a laser, or with topical application of caustic chemical agents.

Condyloma acuminatum, or venereal warts, are usually located on the genital or anal mucosa. These lesions are caused by HPV subtypes 6 and 11. They are seen intraorally with increasing frequency because of changing sexual practices and AIDS. If the clinician suspects condyloma acuminatum, intraoral lesions should be surgically excised. If the diagnosis of condyloma acuminatum is confirmed, the patient's immunologic status and risk for other sexually transmitted diseases must be assessed.

When lesions are diagnosed histopathologically as exhibiting viral characteristics, especially in patients in whom these lesions recur, consideration must be given to determining the phenotype of the etiologic virus. Specimens should be submitted in an appropriate transport medium for in situ hybridization, which will identify the specific HPV subtype present in the tissue. If a diagnosis of an HPV oncovirus is confirmed, long-term patient follow-up is mandatory due to the malignant predisposition of these types of viral lesions.

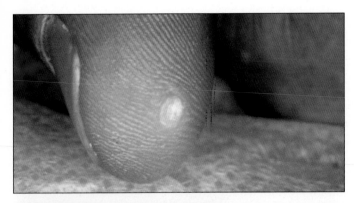

Fig 5-12 Multiple intraoral viral papillomas in a 42-year-old man who habitually chewed the wart from his thumb. No recurrence was noted following surgical removal of the lesions.

Fig 5-12a Cutaneous verruca vulgaris on the thumb.

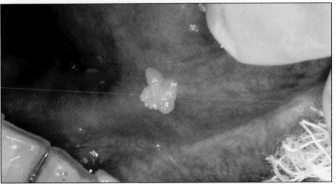

Fig 5-12b Ventral surface of the tongue.

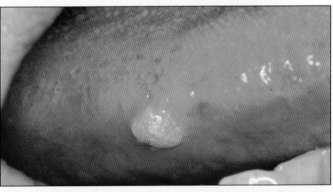

Fig 5-12c Right lateral tongue border.

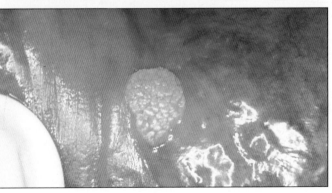

Fig 5-12d Mucosa of the lower lip.

Autoimmune Deficiency Syndrome

Patients with AIDS are at an increased risk of developing oral cancer. These tumors may include, but are not limited to, epidermoid carcinoma, Kaposi's sarcoma, and lymphoma.[25,26] A biopsy should be performed on a persistent mucosal lesion noted in a patient with AIDS to establish the diagnosis.

References

1. Waldron CA, Shaffer WG. Leukoplakia revisited: A clinical immunopathologic study of 3256 oral leukoplakias. Cancer 1975;36:1386–1392.

2. Langlais RP, Miller CS. Color Atlas of Common Oral Diseases, ed 1. Philadelphia: Lea and Febiger, 1992:54–55.

3. Lumerman H, Friedman P, Kerpel S. Oral epithelial dysplasia and the development of invasive squamous carcinoma. Oral Surg Oral Med Oral Pathol Oral Radiol Endod 1995;79:321–329.

4. Shibuya H, Amagasa T, Seto K, Ishibashi K, Horiuchi J, Suzuki S. Leukoplakia-associated multiple carcinomas in patients with tongue carcinoma. Cancer 1986; 57:843–846.

5. Brown RS, Bottomley WK, Abromovich K, Langlais RP. Immediate biopsy versus a therapeutic trial in the diagnosis of vesiculobullous/vesiculoerosive oral lesions. Oral Surg Oral Med Oral Pathol 1992;73:694–697.

6. Abey LM, Kaugers GE, Gunsolley JC, Burns JC, Page DG, Svirsky JA, et al. Intraexaminer and interexaminer reliability in the diagnosis of oral epithelial dysplasia. Oral Surg Oral Med Oral Pathol Oral Radiol Endod 1995;80:188–191.

7. Silverman S Jr, Gorsky M, Lozada F. Oral leukoplakia and malignant transformation: A follow-up study of 257 patients. Cancer 1984;53:563–568.

8. Silverman S Jr. Oral Cancer, ed 4. American Cancer Society. Hamilton, BC: Decker, 1998:36.

9. Shafer WG, Hine MK, Levy BM. A Textbook of Oral Pathology, ed 4. Philadelphia: Saunders, 1983:108.

10. Douglas CW, Gammon MD. Reassessing the epidemiology of lip cancer. Oral Surg Oral Med Oral Pathol 1984;57:631.

11. Manganaro AM, Will MJ, Poulos E. Actinic cheilitis: A premalignant condition. Gen Dent 1997;45:492–494.

12. Lynch MA, Brightman VJ, Greenberg MS. Burket's Oral Medicine, ed 9. Philadelphia: JB Lippincott, 1994: 96–97.

13. Vincent SD, Fotos PG, Baker KA, Williams TP. Oral lichen planus: The clinical, historical, and therapeutic features of 100 cases. Oral Surg Oral Med Oral Pathol 1990;70:165–171.

14. Van Dis ML, Parks ET. Prevalence of oral lichen planus in patients with diabetes mellitus. Oral Surg Oral Med Oral Pathol Oral Radiol Endod 1995;79:696–700.

15. Eisenberg E, Krutchkoff DJ. Lichenoid lesions of the oral mucosa: Diagnostic criteria and their importance in the alleged relationship to oral cancer. Oral Surg Oral Med Oral Pathol 1992;73:699–704.

16. Allen CM. Is lichen planus really premalignant? Oral Surg Oral Med Oral Pathol Oral Radiol Endod 1998;85:347.

17. Silverman S Jr, Gorsky M, Lozada-Nur F. A prospective follow-up study of 570 patients with oral lichen planus: Persistence remission and malignant association. Oral Surg Oral Med Oral Pathol 1985;60:30–34.

18. Silverman S Jr, Gorsky M, Lozada-Nur F, Giannotti K. A prospective study of findings and management in 214 patients with oral lichen planus. Oral Surg Oral Med Oral Pathol 1991;72:665–670.

19. Silverman S Jr, Bahl S. Oral lichen planus update, clinical characteristics, treatment responses, and malignant transformation. Am J Dent 1997;10:259–263.

20. Creath CJ, Cutter G, Bradley DH, Wright TJ. Oral leukoplakia and adolescent smokeless tobacco use. Oral Surg Oral Med Oral Pathol 1991;72:35–41.

21. Connoly GN, Winn DM, Hecht SS, Henningfield JE, Walker B, Hoffmann D. The reemergence of smokeless tobacco. N Engl J Med 1986;314:1020–1027.

22. Hansen LS, Olson JA, Silverman S Jr. Proliferative verrucous leukoplakia. Oral Surg Oral Med Oral Pathol 1985;60:285–298.

23. Silverman S Jr, Gorsky M. Proliferative verrucous leukoplakia: A follow-up study of 54 cases. Oral Surg Oral Med Oral Pathol Oral Radiol Endod 1997;84: 154–157.

24. Miller CS, White DK. Human papillomavirus expression in oral mucosa, premalignant conditions, and squamous cell carcinoma. Oral Surg Oral Med Oral Pathol Oral Radiol Endod 1996;82:57–68.

25. Scully C, Laskaris G, Pindborg J, Porter SR, Reichart P. Oral manifestations of HIV infection and their management. I. More common lesions. Oral Surg Oral Med Oral Pathol 1991;71:158–166.

26. Scully C, Laskaris G, Pindborg J, Porter SR, Reichart P. Oral manifestations of HIV infection and their management. II. Less common lesions. Oral Surg Oral Med Oral Pathol 1991;71:167–171.

CHAPTER 6

Types of Oral Cancer

Robert A. Ord, DDS, MD, MS

Although the most common oral cancer is squamous cell carcinoma, there is a wide variety of primary and secondary malignancies that may occur in the oral cavity. This chapter presents the more frequently seen malignant neoplasms other than squamous cell carcinoma.

Epidermoid Carcinomas

Squamous cell carcinoma is the classic epidermoid carcinoma; however, other epidermoid carcinomas that occur in the oral cavity include verrucous carcinoma, spindle cell carcinoma, basaloid carcinoma, adenosquamous carcinoma, and basosquamous carcinoma.

Verrucous carcinoma lesions typically present as exophytic, cauliflower, or wartlike masses usually associated with leukoplakia (Fig 6-1). Classically they are said to be associated with "snuff dipping." The importance of this cancer is that it is slow-growing and usually grows superficially rather than invading deeply, although the tumor does invade bone rapidly (see Fig 4-1b). It is common on the gingiva, palate, buccal mucosa, and tongue.

Histologically the tumor appears benign with thickened epithelium and bulbous rete pegs with parakeratin-filled clefts. The tumor invades with a pushing rather than an infiltrating front. The diagnosis of cancer may be missed by an inexperienced pathologist or when the biopsy is too shallow, because the cytologic features of malignancy are absent. Both clinically and histologically this cancer may be diagnosed as a papilloma, verrucous hyperplasia, or proliferative verrucous leukoplakia. The tumor shows little tendency to lymph node metastasis, so prognosis is good.[1] However, it is wise to remember that a percentage of these tumors are mixed, showing areas of squamous as well as verrucous carcinoma. These variants behave more aggressively like a true squamous cell carcinoma.[2] In addition, they may occasionally show dedifferentiation to very aggressive anaplastic carcinomas that metastasize rapidly. This change was once thought to occur in relation to irradiation, and previous theory held that these tumors should not be irradiated.[3] However, more recent studies have shown that anaplastic change may occur spontaneously or following surgery, and radiation may be given when indicated.[4] The treatment of choice for this cancer is surgery. Although prognosis is much

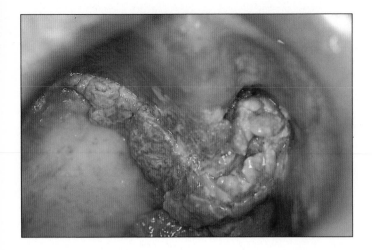

Fig 6-1 Verrucous carcinoma in the left maxillary tuberosity with a typical exophytic warty appearance. The tumor extends across the palate toward the midline.

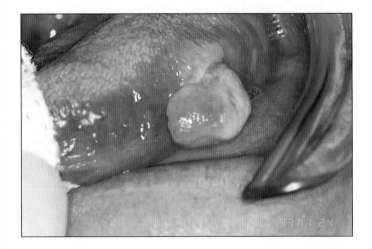

Fig 6-2 Polypoid appearance of spindle cell carcinoma of the tongue. Note associated leukoplakia superiorly.

better than that for squamous cell carcinoma, because of the absence of lymph node involvement anaplastic change is usually fatal, and verrucous carcinoma's occasional widespread involvement of local structures (eg, skull base) may kill the patient.

Spindle cell carcinoma is an uncommon variety of epidermoid carcinoma. This tumor appears as a polypoid lesion of the lip, tongue, or gingiva and may have no surface ulceration (Fig 6-2). The mucosal surface may exhibit only dysplasia, although invasive carcinoma may be present. However, the characteristic malignant spindle cells are seen below the epithelium or dropping off the epithelium. Differential diagnosis includes carcinoma and sarcoma.[5,6] The diagnosis is usually facilitated by immunohistochemical staining for cytokeratin or by electron microscopy. These lesions behave aggressively, with 55% of affected

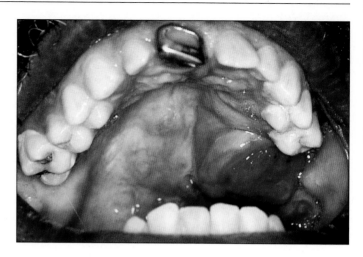

Fig 6-3 Basaloid carcinoma of the maxillary alveolus and antrum in a young man. The patient showed pulmonary metastases within 2 weeks of presentation and died of the disease 6 weeks later.

patients dying and a mean survival time of less than 2 years in one large series.[6] Spindle cell carcinoma may occasionally recur as squamous cell carcinoma and vice versa. The basaloid carcinoma (Fig 6-3), adenosquamous carcinoma, and basosquamous carcinoma are rare varieties of epidermoid carcinoma. All of these tumor types carry a worse prognosis than squamous cell carcinoma with aggressive local growth and early regional metastases.

Salivary Gland Carcinomas

Intraoral, minor salivary gland tumors form 10% to 15% of all salivary gland tumors, and overall approximately 50% of these tumors are malignant. The vast majority of minor salivary gland tumors occur in the palate, usually at the junction of the hard and soft palate to one side of the midline. Only 0.5% to 1% of salivary tumors occur in the sublingual gland, but

more than 90% of these tumors are cancerous.[7] A large number of histologic types of salivary cancers vary from slow-growing, low-grade cancers to very aggressive neoplasms with early metastases. Polymorphous low-grade adenocarcinoma, mucoepidermoid carcinoma, and adenoid cystic carcinoma are typically the most frequently seen.

Polymorphous low-grade adenocarcinoma (PLGA) has been recognized in the past 25 years.[8] Adenocarcinomas as a group have a poor prognosis for survival; however, it has become apparent that PLGA is slow-growing, has little tendency to metastasis, and has an excellent cure rate. The most common site for PLGA is the palate (Fig 6-4). As its name suggests, the tumor can show different patterns, such as solid, tubular, cylindromatous, and Indian file cells, in different areas of the same tumor. Therefore, a biopsy specimen of one area may not be representative and initially PLGA may be wrongly diagnosed, for example, as pleomorphic adenoma or adenoidcys-

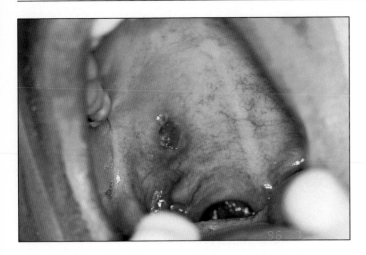

Fig 6-4 Polymorphous low-grade adenocarcinoma.

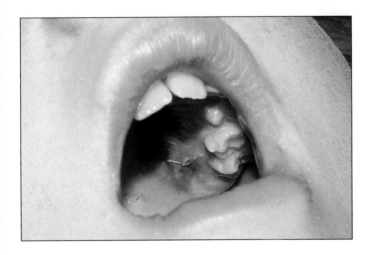

Fig 6-5 A 10-year-old girl with cystic salivary tumor of the palate. The lesion was resected with a 1-cm margin. The patient was alive and well 3 years postoperatively.

tic carcinoma. Although this tumor frequently shows histologic evidence of perineural invasion, this does not seem to be associated with a worse prognosis. This is in marked contrast to most other cancers, such as squamous cell carcinoma or adenoid cystic carcinoma, where perineural invasion significantly reduces the patient's chance of survival. The treatment is conservative excision with a 1-cm margin, including bone if it is involved. These tumors require long-term follow-up because they can recur many years after the original excision.

Lymph node metastasis and distant metastasis are reported but rare. The role of radiation therapy or chemotherapy is not well defined for PLGA.

Mucoepidermoid carcinoma histologically consists of three cell types: squamous cell, intermediate cell, and mucous cell. The greater the number of squamous cells in relation to mucous cells, the more aggressively the tumor behaves. On this basis these tumors are classified as high grade, intermediate grade, and low grade. Fortunately, the low-grade mucoepidermoid carcinoma is the most common type and behaves as a slow-growing cancer that rarely metastasizes.[9] There are several features of this tumor that may, however, disguise its nature as a cancer and lead the dentist to delay diagnosis.

First, because of the high percentage of mucus-producing cells, large cysts may be present in the tumor, which may present as a mucocele in the mouth. However, true mucoceles are very rare in the palate or in the retromolar fossa distal to the mandibular wisdom tooth (a site of prediction for mucoepidermoid carcinoma). Cystic lesions at these sites should be viewed with suspicion. Second, this tumor is the most common salivary cancer in children[10] (Fig 6-5), and any cystic or solid mass in the palate of a child requires biopsy. Third, a proportion of these tumors are interosseous and may present on routine radiographs as odontogenic cysts.

Initial diagnosis of an odontogenic cyst is facilitated with incisional biopsy. Periodic acid–Schiff (PAS) and mucicarmine stains identify the mucous cells and aid the pathologist in histologic diagnosis. The treatment is excision of the tumor with a 1-cm margin of normal tissue.

The high-grade mucoepidermoid carcinoma is an aggressive cancer that readily metastasizes to the cervical nodes and behaves like squamous cell carcinoma (Figs 6-6a to 6-6c).

These cancers require radical surgery combined with radiation therapy. However, the prognosis is frequently poor. Histologically it may be difficult to differentiate these tumors from squamous cell carcinoma; however, PAS or mucicarmine stains show occasional mucous cells. In the author's experience, these tumors are very difficult to cure, frequently metastasizing to the lungs and systemically. They are also relatively radiation resistant.

The adenoid cystic carcinoma is said to be the most common minor salivary gland cancer. It is slow-growing, and patients may have a mass for many years. This slow growth may lull the dentist into a false sense of security that this is a benign lesion and emphasizes the need for biopsy even in long-standing lesions. The author has seen one patient whose denture was fabricated to accommodate her palatal "taurus," which had been noted for 7 years.

Despite its slow growth, adenoid cystic carcinoma is a high-grade lesion, and although 5-year survival is reasonable, survival is poor if patients are observed for 10 years or longer. This tumor is unusual because it will usually metastasize via the bloodstream to the lungs, liver, and bone rather than to the lymph nodes. Histologically the tumor consists of small, darkly staining cells and exhibits tubular, cribriform (Swiss cheese–like), and solid patterns. Tumors with a solid pattern have the worst outlook. Local growth includes perineural spread, which can lead to a tumor well beyond the visible margins. The tumor infiltrates and destroys muscle and bone. Because of its widespread nature (Figs 6-7a and 6-7b), surgery is difficult, requiring large margins. The role of radiation therapy is controversial. Even when lung metastases are present, the patient may live more than 5 years because of the slow growth. The tumor is characterized by its slow, relentless progression with multiple recurrences eventually leading to the death of the patient.

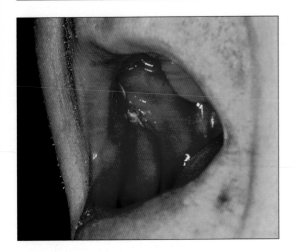

Fig 6-6a Mass in right cheek opposite tuberosity.

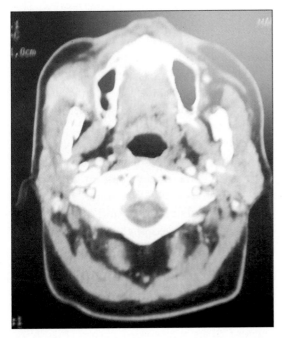

Fig 6-6b Computed tomography (CT) scan showing infiltration into the masseter muscle and temporal space.

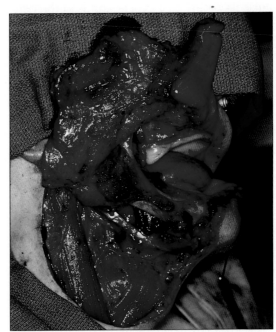

Fig 6-6c Operative photograph of patient showing right supraomohyoid neck dissection, lip split, and cheek flap. This procedure provides access to the masseter and pterygoid region following coronoidectomy.

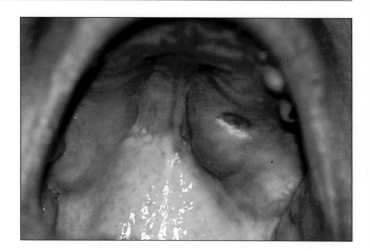

Fig 6-7a Palatal adenoid cystic carcinoma which appears restricted to the oral cavity.

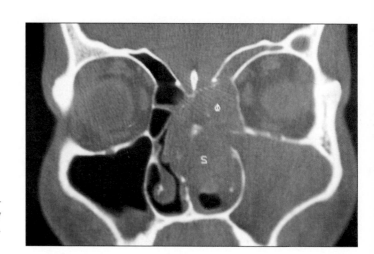

Fig 6-7b CT scan showing widespread involvement of the maxillary sinus, orbital floor, and ethmoid bones.

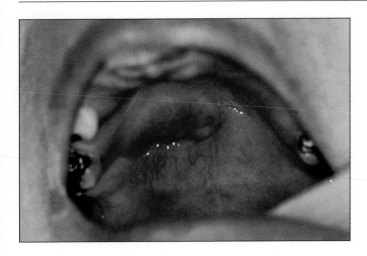

Fig 6-8 Mass at junction of the hard and soft palate resembles a minor salivary gland tumor but is a non-Hodgkins lymphoma.

Lymphomas

Intraoral lymphomas are most common in the region of Waldeyer's ring of lymphatic tissue. This region comprises the lingual tonsil, pharyngeal tonsil, adenoids, and the area at the junction of the hard and soft palate (Fig 6-8). The lesions may be submucosal soft masses with prominent overlying blood vessels, or fast-growing, ulcerated, exophytic lesions resembling carcinomas. Patients may present with enlarged lymph nodes and should always be asked about systemic symptoms (ie, weight loss, night sweats, skin rashes, lumps in the axilla or groin). Patients with HIV are at higher risk of lymphoma development (Fig 6-9). Most of these lymphomas are B-cell non-Hodgkins lymphomas. When lymphoma is suspected, the biopsy material should be sent fresh to enable cytogenetic and flow cytometry tests, which are important in classification and diagnosis. Because lymphoma is a systemic disease, computed tomography scans of the chest and abdomen and bone marrow aspiration are important in depicting other disease sites and staging the lymphoma. Patients require treatment with radiation therapy or chemotherapy.

Unusual Cancers of the Oral Cavity

Virtually any malignant tumor can present in the oral cavity. The main groups of cancers not already discussed are the sarcomas and secondary metastases. In addition, multiple myeloma is well reported.

Sarcomas

These mesenchymal tumors are usually characterized by the presence of malignant spindle cells and their propensity for hematogenous spread. In the oral cavity and jaws, fibrosarcomas, osteosarcomas, chondrosarcomas, liposarcomas, fibrous histiocystomas, neurofibrosarcomas, rhabdomyosarcoma, and angiosarcomas have all been described. Depending on

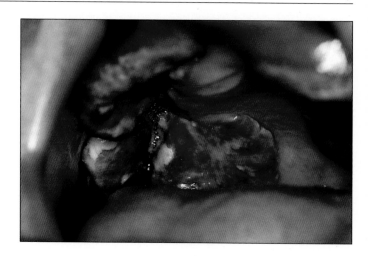

Fig 6-9 Exophytic mass on the maxillary ridge of a patient with HIV. This is a B-cell lymphoma.

their histologic type, treatment may consist of surgery, radiation therapy, or chemotherapy and frequently requires a combination of these modalities. In sarcomas the histologic grade of the tumor is frequently the most important factor determining prognosis.

Rhabdomyosarcoma

Rhabdomyosarcoma is the most common sarcoma of the head and neck in children, and 40% of rhabdomyosarcomas are seen in the head and neck. Rapidly growing, lobulated fleshy tumors in childhood, particularly occurring in the region of the soft palate, should undergo urgent biopsy (Fig 6-10). Treatment is usually based on chemotherapy with surgery and radiation therapy used in combination when indicated. Prognosis is related to the site, stage, and histologic type. Tumors primarily involving the orbit and having an embryonic or botryoid histologic composition have the best outlook; tumors of parameningeal sites or with alveolar or pleomorphic histologic composition have more guarded prognoses.

Osteosarcoma

Osteosarcoma of the jaws is most common in the third decade of life and is much less common than long bone osteosarcoma. The prognosis for jaw tumors is much better than that for osteosarcomas in general, which is presumably related to a decreased tendency to metastasize, and the fact that most jaw osteosarcomas are of the chondroblastic type. The earliest radiological sign is a widening of the periodontal membrane (see Fig 4-2), although radiographs may also show the classic "sunray" appearance (Fig 6-11). The extent of marrow invasion is better delineated with CT or magnetic resonance imaging; an isotope scan is useful in assessing involvement of other bones in addition to the primary site. Computed tomography of the lungs is mandatory to detect metastases. Treatment is by wide surgical excision with good negative margins (Fig 6-12).

The role of chemotherapy for treatment of jaw tumors is less clear than for long bones; however, recent research indicates that chemotherapy should be used.[12]

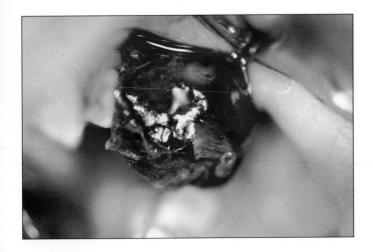

Fig 6-10 Fleshy, hemorrhagic lesion (a rhabdomyosarcoma) growing out of the extraction socket of the second maxillary deciduous molar in a 5-year-old boy.

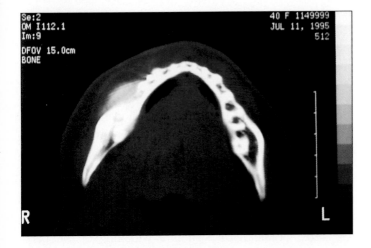

Fig 6-11 CT scan showing "sun ray speckling" buccal to the first molar in a mandibular osteosarcoma.

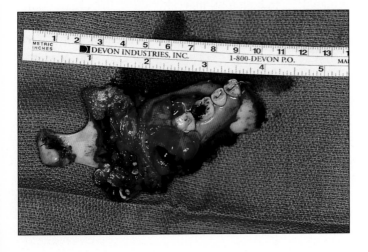

Fig 6-12 Mandibular osteosarcoma in the wisdom tooth region. Resection extends from the condyle to the canine.

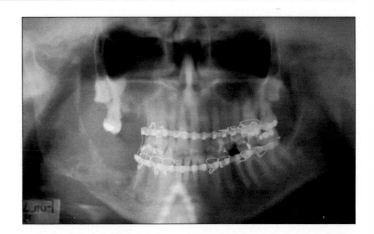

Fig 6-13 Panoramic radiograph showing the widespread moth-eaten appearance of the right mandible with pathologic fracture in a woman with metastatic breast carcinoma.

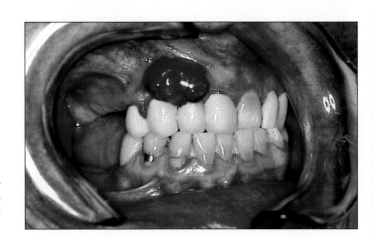

Fig 6-14 Melanoma of the anterior maxilla. Despite radical surgery, the patient died of local recurrence within 6 months.

Metastatic tumors

Although metastases can theoretically involve the jaws from any primary site, the five classic cancers that involve bone are lung, breast, prostate, kidney, and thyroid. The posterior mandible and condyle are the sites most often affected (see Fig 4-3), possibly due to the presence of red marrow in this region. Carcinoma of the kidney is unusual in that it metastasizes more frequently to the maxilla and paranasal sinuses and is hemorrhagic. Metastatic tumors may cause widespread bone destruction and may present with pathologic fractures (Fig 6-

13). Treatment of these lesions is symptomatic and may involve surgical resection, radiation therapy, or chemotherapy.

Melanoma

Mucosal melanoma is rare and carries an ominous prognosis. The site of predilection is the anterior maxilla (Fig 6-14), and it can arise from an area of premalignant melanosis. The lesion may spread to both lymphatics and blood vessels and give rise to rapid dissemination. However, its behavior is unpredictable

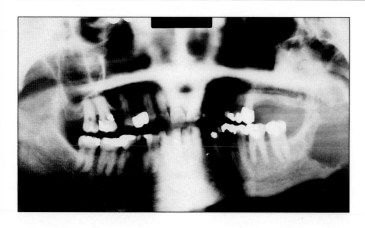

Fig 6-15 A 78-year-old man with previously undiagnosed myeloma presenting with right temporomandibular joint pain due to pathologic fracture.

and occasional spontaneous resolution has been reported. The lesion is relatively radiation resistant, and chemotherapy regimens have proven ineffective to a large degree. Surgery remains the mainstay of therapy, although research into immunotherapy has shown some promising results and melanoma "vaccines" have been developed.

Currently much interest revolves around the technique of sentinel node biopsy, which uses a radioactive isotope to label the lymph node to which the melanoma is most likely to metastasize. Once this lymph node is identified, it is removed and examined histologically. If it is unaffected, then no further neck surgery is required. If it shows metastasis, a neck dissection is undertaken.

Multiple myeloma

Multiple myeloma is a systemic disease and is the most common primary malignant tumor of bone. The lesion is a tumor of plasma cells

characterized by a monoclonal gammaglobulinemia. The bony lesions are usually round and punched out in appearance, while soft tissue involvement is characterized by fleshy swellings. The diagnosis is facilitated by biopsy, serum electrophoresis, and the presence of Bence Jones protein in the urine. Typically the patient presents with lower back pain, and the diagnosis is usually made before jaw lesions appear (Fig 6-15). Treatment includes chemotherapy, and bone marrow transplantation is used increasingly.

Summary

Although squamous cell carcinoma is the most common oral cancer, many other malignant neoplasms can occur in the mouth. Even though a lesion may not look like a typical cancer, if it is persistent and unexplainable, the vigilant dentist should be prepared to perform a biopsy and obtain a histologic diagnosis.

References

1. Batsakis JG, Hybels R, Crissman JD, Rice DH. The pathology of head and neck tumors. Verrucous carcinoma. Head Neck Surg 1982;5:29–38.

2. Medina JE, Dichtel MAJ, Luna MA. Verrucous-squamous carcinomas of the oral cavity: A clinico-pathologic study of 104 cases. Arch Otolaryngol 1984; 10:437–440.

3. Perez CA, Kraus FT, Evans JC, Powers WE. Anaplastic transformation in verrucous carcinoma of the oral cavity after radiation therapy. Radiology 1966;86: 108–115.

4. McDonald JS, Crissmon JD, Gluchman JL. Verrucous carcinoma of the oral cavity. Head Neck Surg 1982;5:22–28.

5. Tse JJ, Aughton W, Zirkin RM, Mermon GE. Spindle cell carcinoma of the oral mucosa: Case report with immunoperoxidase and electron microscopic studies. J Oral Maxillofac Surg 1987;45:267–270.

6. Ellis GL, Corio RL. Spindle cell carcinoma of the oral cavity: A clinicopathologic assessment of fifty-nine cases. Oral Surg Oral Med Oral Pathol 1980;50: 528–534.

7. Ord RA. Management of intra-oral salivary gland tumors. Oral Maxillofac Surg Clin North Am 1994; 6:499–522.

8. Evans MC, Batsakis JG. Polymorphous low-grade adenocarcinoma of minor salivary glands: A study of 14 cases of a distinctive neoplasm. Cancer 1984;53:935.

9. Eversole LR. Muco epidermoid carcinoma: Review of 815 reported cases. J Oral Surg 1470;28:490–496.

10. Krolls SO, Trodhad JN, Boyers RC. Salivary gland lesions in children: A survey of 430 cases. Cancer 1972;30:459–469.

11. Newton WA, Soule EH, Hamunchi AB, et al. Histopathology of childhood sarcomas: Intergroup rhabdomyosarcoma studies I and II: Clinicopathologic correlation. J Clin Oncol 1988;6:67–75.

12. Smeele LE, Kostense PJ, Van der Waul I, Snow GB. Effects of chemotherapy on survival of craniofacial osteosarcoma: A systematic review of 201 patients. J Clin Oncol 1997;15:363–367.

PART II

Management

CHAPTER 7

Surgical Management of Oral Cancer

Robert A. Ord, DDS, MD, MS

General Principles

The management of squamous cell carcinoma depends most importantly on the tumor's stage, although other prognostic factors also influence treatment. At present, squamous cell carcinoma of the oral cavity and jaws is primarily managed with surgery and radiation therapy. Chemotherapy is not a first-line treatment, as prospective trials have not demonstrated increased survival.[1] Chemotherapy combined with radiation therapy has been used in organ-sparing protocols in the larynx, and chemotherapy has been used as an adjunctive therapy in stage IV disease and as a palliative treatment for unresectable disease.

Initial therapy is based on the stage of the cancer. Conventional staging uses the TNM system,[2] in which *T* stands for tumor, *N* for nodes, and *M* for metastases. The T classification is largely dependent on the size of the primary tumor (Table 7-1), whereas the N classification depends on both the size and number of involved nodes (Table 7-2). The M classification is the simplest because tumors are classified as either M0 (ie, show no evidence of distant metastases) or M1 (ie, show evidence

of distant metastases). This classification is then used to divide tumors into stages (Table 7-3), which have prognostic implications. Although overall survival for oral cancer is approximately 50%, in early stage I disease, cure rates are greater than 90%, whereas in late stage IV disease, cure rates are less than 10%. TNM classification and staging is done using the information derived from clinical examination and diagnostic investigations as outlined in chapters 3 and 4.

Although the TNM staging system is widely used to assess prognosis, determine treatment, and compare results from different protocols and centers worldwide, it is by no means perfect. Histologic examination of neck dissection specimens from patients with enlarged lymph nodes thought to be clinically positive may not reveal cancer, and conversely, microscopic cancer may be discovered in lymph nodes that were thought to be normal on palpation and imaging. In these cases the pTNM (staging following pathology, *p*) may be used to restage the tumor. This information is obviously never available in patients treated nonsurgically. In addition, many other factors that significantly impact patient survival (eg, grade of tumor,

Table 7-1	TNM System: T Classification
T	Primary tumor
TX	Primary tumor cannot be assessed
T0	No evidence of primary tumor
Tis	Carcinoma in situ
T1	Tumor 2 cm or less
T2	Tumor greater than 2 cm but not greater than 4 cm
T3	Tumor greater than 4 cm
T4	Tumor invades adjacent structures (eg, through cortical bone, into deep extrinsic muscle of tongue, maxillary sinus, skin)

Table 7-2	TNM System: N Classification
N	Regional lymph nodes
NX	Regional nodes cannot be assessed
N0	No regional lymph node metastasis
N1	Metastasis in a single ipsilateral lymph node, 3 cm or less
N2	
N2a	Metastasis in a single ipsilateral lymph node, greater than 3 cm but not greater than 6 cm
N2b	Metastasis in multiple ipsilateral lymph nodes, none greater than 6 cm
N2c	Metastasis in bilateral or contralateral lymph nodes, none greater than 6 cm
N3	Metastasis in a lymph node greater than 6 cm

Table 7-3	Stage Grouping According to TNM System		
Stage I	T1	N0	M0
Stage II	T2	N0	M0
Stage III	T3	N0	M0
	T1	N1	M0
	T2	N1	M0
	T3	N1	M0
Stage IV	T4	N0, N1	M0
	Any T	N2, N3	M0
	Any T	Any N	M1

tumor thickness, extracapsular spread of cancer outside a lymph node) are not included in the TNM system.[3]

Stage IV disease encompasses a heterogeneous group of patients, some without positive results in lymph nodes, patients with multiple affected lymph nodes who have a much worse prognosis, and patients with distant metastases who die. Although these cases are all "lumped together," they represent very different problems and outcomes.

There are several broad principles that guide the management of the oral cancer patient. In early stage disease—stages I and II—either surgery or radiation therapy gives similar survival statistics. Therefore, treatment depends on the patient's choice, the surgeon's advice, or other factors, such as the patient's age, general medical health, and prognostic factors outside the TNM system. In general, where all other factors are equal, radiation therapy is usually recommended. Approximately one third of patients in whom radiation therapy fails can be salvaged with surgery, while patients in whom primary surgery fails are rarely cured with subsequent radiation therapy. For small cancers where adequate excision is simple and will cause little morbidity, or for small tumors that invade the jaw bones, surgery is usually best.

In stage III and stage IV disease, the best cure rates are obtained with a combination of surgery and radiation therapy. There is little evidence to show that preoperative radiation therapy is better than postoperative radiation therapy.[4] Most surgeons prefer to administer radiation within 6 weeks of surgery completion.[5] When the patient has three or more affected neck nodes, the risk of distant metastasis is high, and the addition of concomitant chemotherapy with radiation therapy should be considered. Although combination therapy increases locoregional control and cure rate, it also increases the complications and patient morbidity.

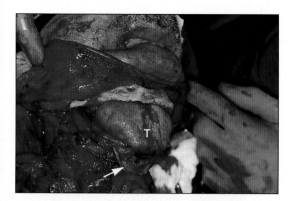

Fig 7-1a The tongue (T), floor of the mouth, and marginal resection of the mandible *(arrow)* pulled through into the neck for excision. The chin and neck flaps are retracted above the lower border of the mandible.

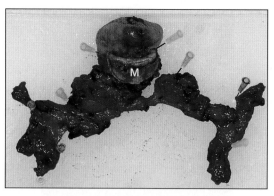

Fig 7-1b Resection specimen with tongue and marginal mandible (M) and bilateral neck dissection.

Principles of Surgery

The surgical objective is to completely remove the primary cancer with any involved cervical lymph nodes, while preserving as many normal structures as possible. The best chance of cure is the first operation, and the surgeon's prime objective is ablation of the cancer, followed by preservation of function, and last, an esthetic result. To achieve these objectives, the surgeon must have excellent access to the tumor, the ability to obtain clear margins, and an understanding of the spread of the tumor to be able to conserve important anatomy.

Surgical access

In small tumors of the anterior floor of the mouth, gingiva, and buccal mucosa, and larger tumors of the mobile oral tongue, an intraoral approach is frequently adequate. When the excision of the primary cancer also involves a neck dissection, the classic surgical teaching is that the primary tumor and neck nodes should be excised in continuity to remove all the lymphatic channels and potential tumor emboli between the primary site and the neck. Evidence exists to support this approach.[6] However, it requires removal of more normal tissue and frequently results in disappointing strands of tissue linking the primary and neck specimens. In cancer of the buccal mucosa and upper gingiva, it is obviously not possible to undertake incontinuity resection.

Small cancers of the mobile tongue are frequently excised separately from any neck dissection. When an incontinuity resection is planned, three approaches are commonly used: the pull-through, the visor, and the mandibular swing. In the pull-through operation, the neck dissection specimen is pedicled to the tissues beneath the primary cancer. The tissues between the primary site and the neck are cut through to form a tunnel between the mouth and the neck. The primary tumor is "pulled through" the tunnel into the neck where it is resected (Figs 7-1a and 7-1b). In anterior tumors, especially where the mandible is to be resected, a tunnel can be made buccal to the mandible via a vestibular

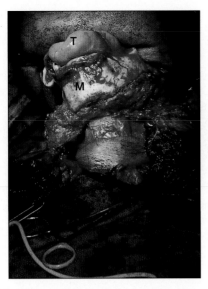

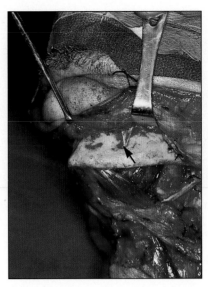

Fig 7-2a The neck flap, soft tissue chin, and lower lip retracted superior to the mandible (M) to allow direct exposure of the jaw and anterior oral cavity. (T = tongue.)

Fig 7-2b Preservation of the mental nerves *(arrow)*.

incision. This allows the neck flaps to be lifted superiorly as a "visor" to expose the mandibular and anterior floor of the mouth (Figs 7-2a and 7-2b).

In large tumors or posterior cancers, such as retromolar fossa carcinomas, the "mandibular swing" approach gives the best access. In this approach the neck contents are pedicled to the tissues beneath the primary tumor. A lip-splitting incision continuous with the neck incision is made (Figs 7-3a to 7-3e). The mandible is exposed buccally and an osteotomy made anterior to the mental foramen. By using periapical radiographs to assess root position and thin bladed saws for the osteotomy cuts, it is usually possible to cut between teeth without having to extract them. Once the lingual tissues are incised, the mandible can be swung laterally to give superb access to the oral cavity (Figs 7-4a and 7-4b). The infe-

rior alveolar nerve is preserved, and the mandible is replaced following tumor resection and fixed with plates (Fig 7-3). The development of plates for the craniofacial region has allowed rigid fixation of bony osteotomies, preserving facial bones, and has led to the development of a variety of transfacial approaches to skull base tumors.

Surgical margins

The objective of having good surgical access is to allow the surgeon to obtain the requisite safe margins for complete excision of the cancer. In most cases this will be a minimum of 1 cm in all directions, including depth (Fig 7-5).[7] The excision is monitored by frozen sections taken at surgery. However, the true margins can only be assessed on the final speci-

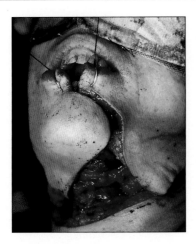

Fig 7-3a The lip-split incision carried around the submental fold and chin prominence for better final esthetics.

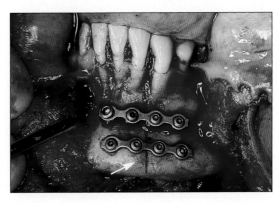

Fig 7-3b Osteotomy cut *(arrow)* marked between the mandibular left canine and lateral incisor. Plates are placed prior to completing the osteotomy, then removed.

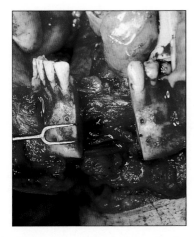

Fig 7-3c Retraction of the osteotomized mandible allowing access to the deep anterior floor of the mouth in a case of sublingual gland cancer.

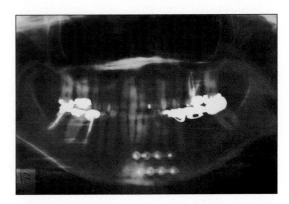

Fig 7-3d Postoperative panoral radiograph showing placement of plates to put the mandible back in its original position.

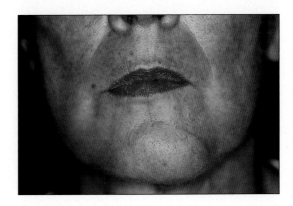

Fig 7-3e Six months postsurgery. Careful suturing and alignment of the soft tissues allow a good esthetic result.

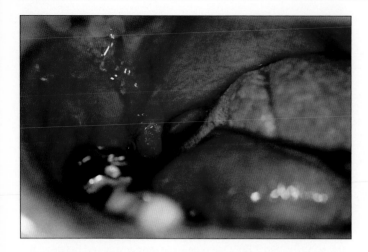

Fig 7-4a Retromolar fossa carcinoma ideally approached via a mandibular swing osteotomy.

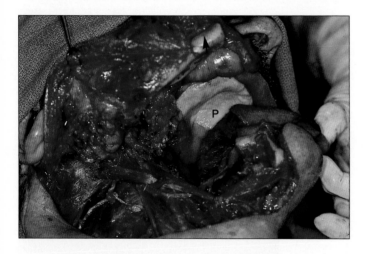

Fig 7-4b Superb access with the mandible *(arrow)* swung superlaterally. (P = palate.)

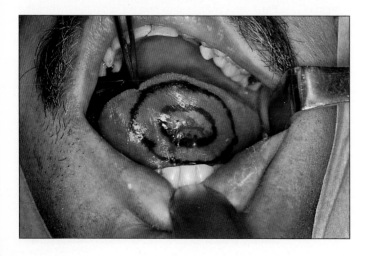

Fig 7-5 Cancer of the tongue with a 1-cm margin marked for resection.

men. If margins are positive for cancer, the patient will either require re-excision or radiation therapy. There are conflicting reports on the efficacy of radiation therapy in the sterilization of residual microscopic disease.[8,9] Recent work on immunostaining p53 in oral cancer has shown that residual cancer cells can be identified in margins that were apparently normal on light microscopy, which may explain why cancers can recur locally despite clear margins.[10] Where nerve trunks (eg, the lingual nerve) are closely associated with the cancer or there is clinical evidence of nerve invasion (tongue cancer with pain radiating to the ear), the nerve is sacrificed. Because squamous cell carcinoma can travel easily along perineural spaces, the nerve is usually followed proximally toward the skull base before sectioning. Frozen section specimens of the cut nerve are sent to the pathologist to confirm clearance of the carcinoma.

Conservative ablation

Although the surgeon's main objective is the elimination of all cancer cells, whenever oncologically feasible, functional tissue should be preserved to aid in rehabilitation. In the past the mandible was frequently unnecessarily sacrificed for access or ablation. Despite improved reconstruction techniques (see chapter 8), it is always best to preserve the patient's mandible, unless this is not possible due to direct cancer invasion.

Improved understanding of the way in which squamous cell carcinoma invades the mandible from the occlusal surface[11] and the histologic patterns of bone invasion allow the surgeon to use marginal resection in early bone invasion.[12] In this technique only the dentoalveolar portion of the mandible is excised, preserving the lower border (Figs 7-6a and 7-6b). This keeps mandibular shape

and continuity. In properly assessed cases, there is no increase in cancer recurrence.[13,14] This technique is most valuable in the curved anterior symphisis region, which is difficult to reconstruct. By excising only the dentoalveolar portion of the mandible, sufficient bone remains to allow denture reconstruction or the placement of implants (Fig 7-6c). In cases where segmental resection of the mandible is required in the body or angle region, it has become apparent that the posterior border of the vertical ramus and condyle are rarely tumorigenic. This allows the surgeon to design osteotomies to remove the invaded mandible and the inferior alveolar nerve that are at risk, while preserving the temporomandibular joint for reconstruction (Figs 7-7a to 7-7c).

Perhaps the area that has changed most dramatically in recent years is the surgical approach to the neck. Crile[15] described the radical neck dissection in 1906 and it remained the standard method for more than 60 years. The surgery is a dissection of all five levels of cervical lymph nodes and was therefore radical, but it gave rise to considerable morbidity because of the removal of the accessory nerve, sternocleidomastoid muscle, and internal jugular vein (Fig 7-8). On the basis of anatomic studies of the cervical fascia, it became accepted that either one, two, or all three of these structures could be preserved with the same oncologic outcome, unless they were directly invaded by tumor.[16] These surgeries were called *modified radical neck dissections* because they still removed all five levels of cervical lymph nodes but preserved structures that would have been sacrificed.

The next advance was the concept that in early neck disease all five levels might not require removal. These neck dissections are known as *selective neck dissections*. The most commonly used procedure for oral cavity cancer is the supraomohyoid neck dissection.[17]

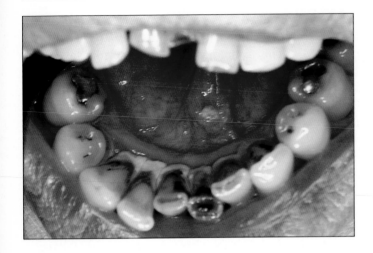

Fig 7-6a Early stage floor of the mouth cancer fixed to lingual perioteum.

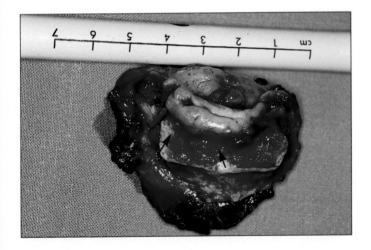

Fig 7-6b Specimen showing marginal resection of the mandible *(arrow).*

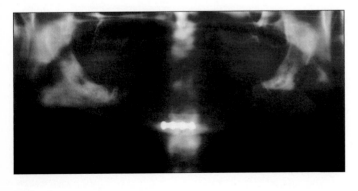

Fig 7-6c Postoperative radiograph showing adequate bone preserved for implant placement anteriorly.

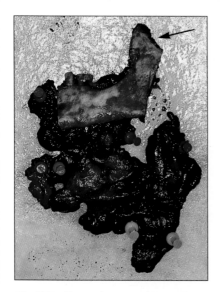

Fig 7-7a Resection specimen showing segmental mandibular resection via subsigmoid osteotomy, removing the coronoid *(arrow)* but preserving the condyle and posterior ramus.

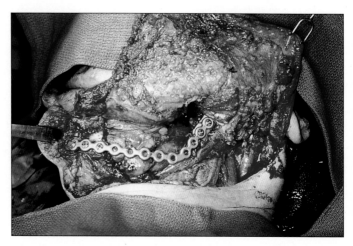

Fig 7-7b Osteotomy allowing immediate placement of a reconstruction bar to restore mandibular continuity and function.

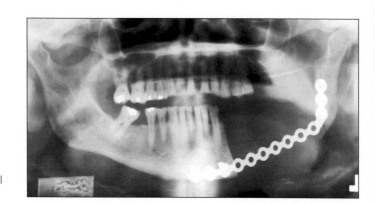

Fig 7-7c Radiograph showing typical postoperative result.

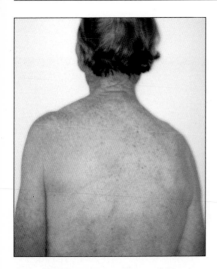

Fig 7-8 Shoulder droop following removal of the accessory nerve in neck dissection.

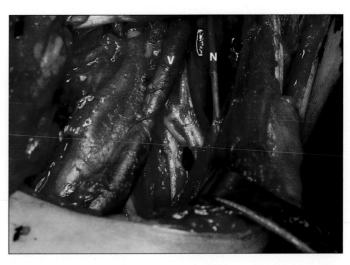

Fig 7-9 Sternocleidomastoid muscle retracted to show internal jugular vein (V) and accessory nerve (N).

This method removes the upper three levels of cervical lymph nodes (ie, the nodes lying superior to the point that the supraomohyoid muscle crosses the internal jugular vein). Included in this dissection are the submandibular and submental triangles, the anterior triangle of the neck, the superior and middle jugular lymph nodes, and the lymph nodes posterosuperior to the accessory nerve. These are the sentinel lymph nodes, which are the nodes primarily affected by oral cancer. All the important structures in the neck are preserved (Fig 7-9). The supraomohyoid neck dissection is primarily used for patients with no palpable lymph nodes and no affected lymph nodes on computed tomography or magnetic resonance imaging, but with a high chance of having occult microscopic nodal metastasis. Patients with large T2, T3, or T4 primary tumors; with tumors thicker than 4 to 5 mm; or with tumors with perineural invasion are known to have more than a 20% chance of occult metastasis.[18,19] It is also important to evaluate other fac-

tors, such as histologic differentiation and a high-risk site (eg, the tongue), when deciding whether to proceed with an elective supraomohyoid neck dissection in the patient with no clinical evidence of cervical disease.

The modern trend is to be aggressive with selective neck dissections in patients with significant risk of lymph node involvement. The supraomohyoid neck dissection has a low morbidity and gives an excellent esthetic outcome (Figs 7-10a and 7-10b). In patients found to have microscopic disease, either a radical neck dissection is scheduled or radiation therapy is administered. In patients who present with advanced neck disease, radical and modified radical neck dissection with postoperative radiation therapy is the standard approach. When the reconstructive surgeon contemplates using a microvascular-free flap, the ablative surgeon attempts to preserve vessels in the neck for flap anastamosis.

In recurrent disease, particularly following radiation therapy, surgery is much more diffi-

Fig 7-10 Good esthetic appearance following bilateral supraomohyoid neck dissection.

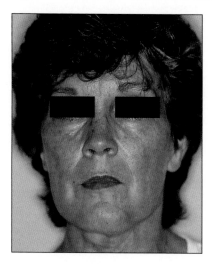

Fig 7-10a Frontal view.

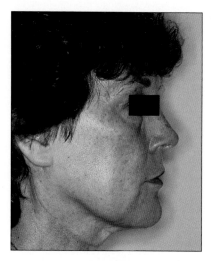

Fig 7-10b Profile view.

cult. The pattern of tumor invasion is more diffuse, and tumor margins are harder to assess. Conservative surgery is less applicable in these cases, because wide excision with sacrifice of any structure that may be involved is usually required. The trend in reconstructive surgery is for immediate reconstruction at ablation. It is usually appropriate to have two separate teams of surgeons so that the ablative surgeon does not "cheat" on the surgical margin because he or she is thinking about the reconstructive defect.

Summary

Surgery, along with radiation therapy, remains the foundation of successful oral cancer treatment. Complete tumor ablation is essential for success. Modern access techniques have allowed the surgeon much more freedom to

excise the tumor with an adequate margin, while being confident that reconstructive surgeons can repair the defect. In addition, a better understanding of the ways in which oral cancer spreads allows preservation of normal structures, which is important in the final functional and esthetic result.

References

1. Fu KK. Combined-modality therapy for head and neck cancer. Oncology 1997;11:1781–1790.

2. Union International Contre Cancer (UICC). TNM, Classification of Malignant Tumors, ed 4. Berlin: Springer Verlag, 1987.

3. MacIntosh RB. Classification and staging of oral cancer. Oral Maxillofac Surg Clin North Am 1997;9: 283–298.

4. Snow JB, Gelbert RD, Kramer S, Davis LW, Marcial VA, Lowry LD. Comparison of pre-operative and postoperative therapy for patients with carcinoma of the head and neck. Acta Otolaryngol 1981;91:11.

5. Vikram B, Strong EW, Shah J, Spiro RH. Elective post-operative radiation therapy in stages III and IV epidermoid carcinoma of the head and neck. Am J Surg 1980;140:580.

6. Leemans CR, Tiwari R, Natua JJP, Snow GB. Discontinuous vs incontinuity neck dissection in carcinoma of the oral cavity. Arch Otolaryngol Head Neck Surg 1991;117:1003–1006.

7. Ord RA, Aisner S. Accuracy of frozen sections in assessing margins in oral cancer resection. J Oral Maxillofac Surg 1997;55:663–669.

8. Mantravadi RVP, Haas E, Liebner EJ, Skolnik EM, Applebaum EL. Post-operative radiotherapy for persistent tumor at the surgical margins in head and neck cancers. Laryngoscope 1983;93:1337.

9. Zieski LA, Johnson JT, Myers EN, Thearle PB. Squamous cell carcinoma with positive margins: Surgery and post-operative radiation. Arch Otolaryngol Head Neck Surg 1986;112:863–866.

10. Brennan JA, Mao L, Hruban RH, et al. Molecular assessment of histopathological staging in squamous cell carcinoma of the head and neck. N Engl J Med 1995;332:429.

11. McGregor AD, MacDonald AG. Routes of entry of squamous cell carcinoma to the mandible. Head Neck Surg 1988;10:294–301.

12. Muller H, Slootweg PJ. Mandibular invasion by oral squamous cell carcinoma: Clinical aspects. J Craniomaxillofac Surg 1990;18:80–84.

13. Dubner S, Heller KS. Local control of squamous cell carcinoma following marginal and segmental mandiblectomy. Head Neck 1993;15:29.

14. Ord RA, Samardi M, Papadimitrou J. A comparison of segmental and marginal bony resection for oral squamous cell carcinoma involving the mandible. J Oral Maxillofac Surg 1997;55:470–477.

15. Crile G. Excision of cancer of the head and neck with special reference to the plan of dissection based on one hundred and thirty-two operations. JAMA 1987;258:3286–3293.

16. Bocca E, Pignataro O. A conservative technique in radical neck dissection. J Laryngol Otol 1966;80:831–838.

17. Medina JE, Byers RM. Supraomohyoid neck dissection: Rationale, indications and surgical technique. Head Neck 1989;11:111–122.

18. Shah JP, Anderson PE. Evolving role of modifications in neck dissection for oral squamous carcinoma. Br J Oral Maxillofac Surg 1995;33:3–8.

19. Ord RA. Current concepts in managing the neck in squamous cell carcinoma of the oral cavity. Oral Maxillofac Surg Clin North Am 1997;9:385–396.

CHAPTER 8

Contemporary Principles of Surgical Reconstruction of the Oral Cavity

Remy H. Blanchaert, Jr, MD, DDS

Resection of oral cancers typically results in the creation of significant three-dimensional defects. Resection may include the tongue, soft tissue lining of the oral cavity, teeth, and bone. Adequate surgical therapy requires the excision of the diseased tissue as well as a margin of tissue that appears healthy, because cancers can invade deeply into adjacent structures. In recent years major advances have been made in the reconstruction of oral cavity, oral pharynx, maxillary, and mandibular defects. Many of these advances are a result of developments in the use and increasing application of free tissue transfer. Significant improvements in function and esthetics following resection have been documented. Reconstruction of defects resulting from complications related to radiation therapy are discussed separately (see chapter 12).

Early attempts at surgical ablation of oral cancers were often associated with primary closure of the resultant defect, which often resulted in severe restriction of mobility, disfigurement, and loss of function. Numerous methods using a variety of flaps have been designed to overcome these problems. This chapter will discuss those techniques that

have proven most useful, provide an understanding of the method of flap selection, and demonstrate results of typical cases.

For rehabilitation of the oral cavity to be complete, replacement of the dentition is mandatory. The role and timing of the placement of dental implants in maxillofacial reconstruction following ablative cancer surgery is discussed as well. The commonly used flaps that have been selected for discussion are the traditional pedicled flap (temporalis, pectoralis major, and latissimus dorsi) and free microvascular flap (radial forearm, rectus abdominus, fibula, and iliac). The head and neck surgeries most often encountered involve mandibulectomy defects, maxillectomy defects, glossectomy defects, and defects resulting from excision of the oral lining tissues (floor of the mouth, pharyngeal wall, and cheek).

Patient Assessment

Preoperative evaluation and assessment of the patient is critical to the success of maxillofacial reconstruction. Only after completely understanding the clinical problem can the reconstructive surgeon contemplate the intricacies of the resultant defect site and devise a suitable reconstruction. The method of reconstruction depends on patient factors (comorbidity, especially peripheral vascular disease), the characteristics of the tumor (size, location, tissues involved, prognosis), and experience of the reconstructive surgeon. The method of reconstruction selected must provide the greatest benefit with the least associated morbidity.

During the planning stage, the reconstructive surgeon develops a primary and secondary plan. Occasionally, the resection extends beyond the boundaries of what was expected upon initial evaluation, or recipient vessels are not available for anastamosis, requiring modification of the treatment plan. The preoperative evaluation is complete only after selecting a primary reconstructive technique and one or two back-up techniques, should complications or difficulty arise.

In recent years the use of free tissue transfer has increased dramatically. The increased technical demands of microsurgery give the impression of increasing health care expenditures. However, this has proven to be false. Brown et al,[1] in a matched-pair analysis, provided an excellent comparison of the role of free tissue transfer in head and neck surgery. They demonstrated that free tissue transfer, although it requires increased operating time, results in comparable expenditures in resources but with improved functional and esthetic results for the patient. Major savings were seen though,

because of decreased hospital stay and fewer complications, such as fistula formation. Al Qattan et al[2] and Singh et al[3] have detailed complications associated with microsurgical head and neck reconstruction and identified factors associated with complications. Kroll et al[4] demonstrated that immediate free flap reconstruction of mandibular defects was associated with significant cost savings and decreased rates of complication compared to the traditional technique of delayed free bone grafting.

Mandibular Reconstruction

Case study: Figure 8-1 demonstrates many of the important principles of primary mandibular reconstruction. The patient presented with advanced squamous cell carcinoma of the floor of the mouth. The tumor had invaded the anterior portions of the tongue and the mandible. The mandible was involved from the left posterior body to the right parasymphysis. Harvest of the free fibula flap was carried out at the same time as the resection to limit operating time. The flap was inset completely prior to revascularization. Key features of the reconstruction are primary restoration of mandibular continuity with well-vascularized bone, and reconstruction of the anterior floor of the mouth with a mobile soft tissue flap that allows movement of the residual tongue.

Fig 8-1 (a) A composite resection of the mandible, floor of the mouth, and tongue with a bilateral neck dissection. (b) A rigid reconstruction is used for restoration of mandibular continuity. (c) The fibula osteoseptocutaneous donor site is outlined with a marker. (d) The skin is soft and pliable, allowing freedom of movement of the tongue base, and the bone can be osteotomized to fit the natural contour of the mandible. The skin receives its blood supply in this case from perforating vessels that travel in the lateral intramuscular septum. A rich network of anastomosing blood vessels exists within the skin and fascia. Occasionally, these vessels traverse the muscle to reach the skin. Their identification and preservation is therefore mandatory. (e) Isolation of the vascular pedicle is seen here. The peroneal artery and the largest of the two veins are identified within the vessel loops near their junction with the posterior tibial artery. (f) The osteoseptocutaneous flap has been harvested. (g) A similar case demonstrates contouring of the bone accomplished with multiple osteotomies prior to revascularization. Note the vascular pedicle just below the inferior border of the mandible.

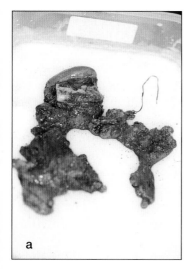

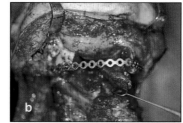

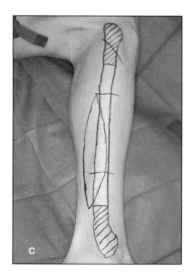

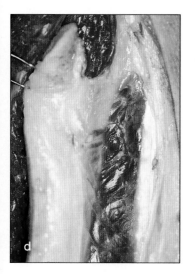

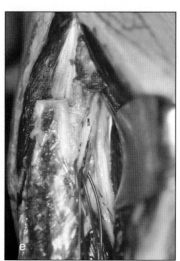

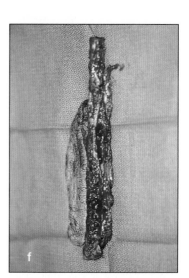

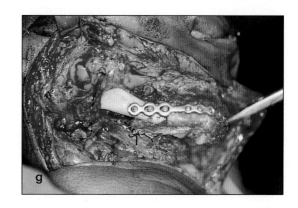

Resection of the mandible is associated with significant disability and deformity. The continuity of the mandible is responsible for protection of the airway in two ways. First, the mandible is a site of insertion for the suprahyoid musculature, which contributes to the elevation of the larynx, preventing aspiration on swallowing. Second, the mandible supports the anterior position of the tongue, which is necessary for the maintenance of an oral airway. With rare exception,[5] the literature supports the primary microvascular flap reconstruction of the mandible as the method most likely to achieve an adequate result. A number of factors favor primary reconstruction, such as less tissue retraction secondary to scarring and fibrosis, fewer hospitalizations, and decreased complications.[6,7]

Primary mandibular reconstruction is best accomplished with free tissue transfer; otherwise the complication rate is unacceptably high. Komisar et al[8] reported infection in four of seven immediate reconstructions using free bone grafting and reconstruction plates. They subsequently documented hospitalization rates for delayed mandibular reconstruction with free bone grafts three times greater than that of patients not undergoing mandibular reconstruction. In another study, Komisar[9] found that improved cosmesis was the only significantly improved factor following delayed bone grafting of the mandible. Careful analysis identified that scarring and fibrosis related to the delayed nature of the reconstruction, as well as a high infection rate, contributed to the poor outcome seen with this technique.

An excellent prospective study by Wagner et al[7] compares presurgical and postsurgical measurements of speech, swallowing, occlusal force, and oral intake in a cohort of patients undergoing segmental mandibulectomy as part of their required oral cancer therapy. Although the study was limited because no nonreconstruction group was analyzed, several impor-

tant predictive parameters were identified. The extent of tongue and pharynx resection, the size of the skin paddle of the bone containing flap, and a diagnosis of malignant disease predicted a worse posttreatment outcome. A plateau of improvement was observed at approximately 3 months following surgery for all parameters except occlusal force, which continued to increase in the 1 year of follow-up.

A controlled study of 10 patients undergoing primary microvascular mandibular reconstruction and 10 patients who did not undergo reconstruction was reported by Urken et al.[6] They documented clear benefits in the group of patients undergoing primary mandibular reconstruction with respect to cosmesis, deglutition, oral competence, speech, length of hospitalization, dental rehabilitation, and general well-being.

Primary free tissue transfer (microvascular flap) mandibular reconstruction is most often undertaken using either the fibula osteoseptocutaneous flap[10] based on the peroneal vessels, or the iliac flap[11-13] based on the deep circumflex iliac vessels. The iliac flap can be designed to include separate paddles of both skin and the internal oblique muscle.

Urken et al[14] reported the experience of one surgeon with 210 cases of vascularized oromandibular free tissue reconstruction. A total of 137 iliac flaps and 46 fibula flaps were presented. An additional 30 cases used two simultaneous free flaps (a bone containing flap and a radial forearm flap). Primary reestablishment of mandibular continuity was successful in 202 patients (96%). Sixteen patients underwent reexploration for vessel-related complications resulting in salvage of one half of that group. This report also documented the primary placement of osseointegrated implants in 81 patients (360 fixtures), providing the largest series of this particular use of dental implants published. The overall success rate of the implants was 92%. In the setting of postoperative radiation therapy, the implant success rate was 86%. Implantation of previously irradiated bone resulted in a success rate of only 64%, although this comprised a very small (14 fixtures) group.

Shpitzer et al[15] provided an analysis of their experience with 50 consecutive mandibular reconstructions using fibula osteoseptocutaneous flaps. The authors concluded that the fibula is an ideal donor site based on length, cortical bone density, anatomy of the blood supply, ability to include a soft tissue paddle, and location, which allowed a two-team surgical procedure. Further support of the fibula flap in mandibular reconstruction has been published. Wolff et al[16] provided an analysis of 24 cases. Lydiatt et al[17] reported 64 cases, 14 of which were in patients who had prior failed attempts at mandibular reconstruction. Chang et al[18] emphasized the primary placement of osseointegrated dental implants.

The iliac composite (skin, muscle, bone) flap is particularly applicable to the reconstruction of extensive composite defects of the oral cavity, mandible, and facial skin. Urken et al[19] documented 10 such cases in a useful report that contains excellent descriptions of flap design and surgical technique.

Regardless of the type of free bone flap selected, the preferred method of establishment of mandibular continuity and premorbid contour is the same. Generally, a rigid reconstruction bar is fashioned and connected to the mandible by placing appropriate length screws proximal and distal to the planned mandibulectomy bone cuts prior to resection. The bar is then removed temporarily and replaced following completion of the resection. In this manner the contour of the mandible is ensured. At the time of flap inset, closing osteotomies (fibula) or opening osteotomies (iliac) are made to allow passive adaptation of the bone flap to the bar. The soft tissue inset is completed after the bone is sta-

bilized to the reconstruction bar. An alternative technique uses several miniplates often placed at right angles to one another across osteotomy sites. This technique could be considered much more difficult.

Futran et al[20] reviewed 95 cases of vascularized bone transfer. The technique already described was used in all of the cases. No plate fractures were seen in the study group. Rapid formation of complete bone union between the native mandible and the bone flap is responsible for the lack of nonunion and resultant plate fracture. Three plates became exposed following mandibular reconstruction. The plates used at that time were of a different configuration than those currently used. (Increasingly, the mandibular plating systems have become lower in profile, resulting in less tension in the overlying facial and neck skin and will likely result in fewer cases of plate exposure.) Similar results were seen in Shpitzer et al,[15] who reviewed 50 cases of vascularized mandibular reconstruction.

An additional advantage of mandibular plating is the potential for in situ modification of the bone flap prior to transection of the vascular pedicle. Chang et al[18] described sterilization of the reconstruction bar after its adaptation, allowing transfer of the plate to the bone flap harvest site. The authors completed all of the necessary osteotomies, as described previously, using a sterile back table to place osseointegrated implants prior to flap inset. They documented their results in 12 patients.

Not all patients are candidates for primary mandibular reconstruction. Peripheral vascular disease, radical neck dissection, or the presence of major comorbidities may preclude free tissue transfer. Likewise, failure of a planned free tissue transfer mandibular reconstruction may require the use of another reconstruction technique. In such instances, a rigid reconstruction bar with or without a pedicled regional myocutaneous flap can be used. Such an approach has an excellent record of success in the lateral and ramus portions of the mandible. Increasing rates of plate exposure and fracture are seen when such a technique must be used in the anterior mandible.

Nonvascularized mandibular reconstruction is generally performed using a rigid reconstruction bar designed to withstand the forces of mastication. Such designs are currently in the third generation of modifications. These plate systems were developed to transfer the load to the interface between the plate and the screw—a significant advantage over the traditional bone plate that bears load at the interface between the plate and the bone. A common result of load transfer between plate and bone is bone resorption with resultant screw loosening and hardware failure. An additional advantage of the newer designs is a lower, smoother profile, which results in fewer instances of plate exposure.

Soft tissue defects associated with composite resection of the mandible are generally obliterated with the pectoralis major myocutaneous flap. This flap has a robust blood supply, following elevation from the anterior chest wall which consists of the thoracicoacromial artery and the lateral thoracic artery. The flap was first described in 1979 by Ariyan.[21] The pectoralis major flap rapidly gained popularity and remains an extremely versatile modality in head and neck reconstruction. Although in the original description by Ariyan the thoracicoacromial artery was the only vessel included, anatomic studies by others[22-24] have resulted in greater appreciation for the role of the lateral thoracic artery in the viability of the pectoralis major myocutaneous flap. The author routinely strives to include this vessel in the flap pedicle. Kiyokawa et al[25] described further modification in the development of the flap. The authors reported excellent results with improved flap blood flow by skeletoniza-

tion of the vascular pedicle and release of the periosteum of the clavicle, allowing an increased arch of rotation by passing the flap beneath the clavicle.

Maxillary Reconstruction

Case study: Figure 8-2 shows an advanced, poorly differentiated adenocarcinoma of the palate. The tumor involved the entire maxilla and the majority of the soft palate. This particular case was not well suited for obturation with a prosthesis because of inadequate retention, and resection of a large portion of the soft palate was required. A rectus abdominus myocutaneous free flap allowed primary obliteration and reconstruction of the defect. The skin portion of the flap was designed to fit precisely the shape of the mucosal defect. The muscle component was used to fill the dead space of the maxillary sinus, to line the lateral wall of the nose, and to add bulk to the soft palate. Following completion of the flap inset, the microvascular anastomosis was completed using the temporal artery and vein as recipient vessels.

Restoration of form to the maxilla following resection has always been a particularly difficult task. Standard therapy consists of a prosthesis (obturator) that requires attachment to adjacent residual teeth for stability. Maintenance of a prosthesis by the edentulous patient is rather tricky. The prosthodontist makes use of existing scar bands to assist in the stabilization of the prosthesis. Air and fluid leaks are common. Frequent adjustments and remakes of the prosthesis are necessary. Because of these significant drawbacks, immediate reconstruction of the maxillectomy defect is desirable. The rectus abdominus

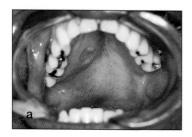

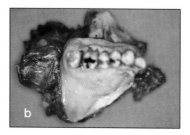

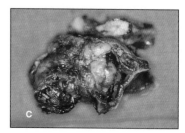

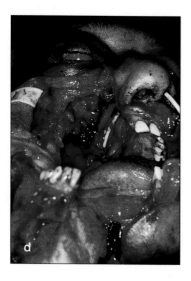

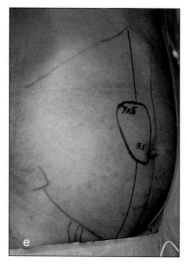

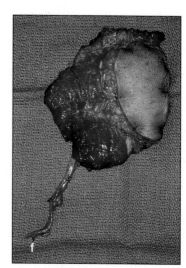

Fig 8-2 (a) A large tumor involving the hard palate. Imaging and palpation reveal that the tumor has invaded the majority of the soft palate and lateral pharyngeal wall. (b,c) The resection specimen shows the extent of the tumor. (d) Note the three-dimensional nature of the resection deformity. (e) The rectus abdominus myocutaneous free flap is outlined on the abdomen. The skin paddle is designed to accommodate the dimensions of the mucosal defect. (f) Additional muscle is harvested to obliterate the sinus, line the nose, and add bulk to the soft palate reconstruction. The deep inferior epigastric vascular pedicle is seen entering the undersurface of the rectus muscle on its lateral border. Careful design of the flap allows acceptable vascular pedicle geometry, avoiding problems with kinking of the small vessels. Recipient vessels for vascular anastomosis are therefore selected prior to design of the flap. (g) The vascular anastomosis is completed to the superficial temporal vessels.

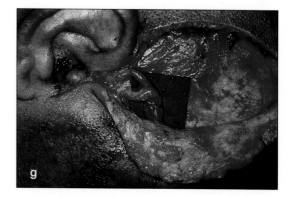

myocutaneous free flap with or without free bone grafting and the iliac flap with internal oblique muscle are two methods by which immediate reconstruction can be accomplished reliably. Previous reports also document the utility of the subscapular system of flaps for maxillary reconstruction.[26]

Careful preoperative patient evaluation and assessment is especially critical in maxillary reconstruction. Magnetic resonance imaging and computed tomographic imaging are essential adjuncts to physical examination to determine the extent of disease spread into adjacent structures (eg, pterygomaxillary space, infratemporal space, orbit, and paranasal sinuses). Palpation of the soft palate provides the reconstructive surgeon with the best appreciation of disease spread. After gaining an adequate appreciation for the anticipated deformity, the reconstruction is planned.

Reconstruction of the underlying contour of the malar prominence and restoration of orbital volume often require free bone grafting with split calvaria. An ideal maxillary reconstruction achieves three major goals: restoration of facial form (support for the orbital contents, cheek, and lip), separation of the nasal cavity from the oral cavity, and creation of a suitable environment for dental rehabilitation.

The superficial temporal artery and vein often serve as recipient vessels for free flap maxillary reconstruction. The proximity of the vessels is excellent, especially following transfacial access to the tumor. Excluding prior surgery in the proximity of the vessels or giant cell arteritis, these vessels are of acceptable quality for either the iliac or the rectus flap. The facial artery and vein are also acceptable recipient vessels.[27] It is best to begin preparation of the free flap only after clearance of surgical margins, necessary bone grafting, and identification and preparation of suitable recipient vessels. The three-dimensional geometry of maxillary reconstruction means minor

deviations from the preoperative surgical plan can result in the need for significant alteration in the design of the flap or the flap pedicle.

Brown[27] reported his conceptualization for maxillary defects and his methods for orientation of the ilium to achieve appropriate facial form (lip support, malar projection). He described the rapid epithelialization and contraction of the internal oblique muscle and cautioned against the use of this flap alone when mobile portions of the soft palate are resected because of immobility and contraction of soft tissue associated with this type of reconstruction. In such a setting, a separate radial forearm flap or temporalis flap is suitable. Likewise, a flap with significantly more bulk, such as the rectus abdominus myocutaneous flap, might prove to be a better reconstruction technique. Brown also described the use of the ipsilateral ilium for the development of the flap. The vessel anastomosis was most often completed at the point where the vessels cross the inferior border of the mandible. Other authors have provided valuable descriptions of the flap harvest technique.[13,28,29]

The rectus abdominus myocutaneous free flap is particularly useful in the reconstruction of extensive maxillectomy defects. The blood supply to the rectus abdominus muscle and the overlying skin has been well described.[30] The preponderance of the musculocutaneous perforators near the umbilicus and their oblique course allow for the development of a flap with muscle oriented in one direction and a skin paddle oriented in another.[31] This is particularly useful in the reconstruction of complex defects with multiple dimensions, as is commonly encountered in maxillectomy defects.[32–34] The rectus muscle is oriented toward the skull base, nasal cavity, and nasal pharynx. It can also be placed adjacent to free bone grafts used in the restoration of the floor of the orbit and zygoma. The muscle is rapidly epithelialized. The skin paddle is oriented toward the mouth and inset into the mucosal defect, providing a watertight and airtight seal.

Kyutoku et al,[32] in their work on orbitofacial reconstruction, documented the excellent outcome of the combination of the rectus flap and vascularized hard tissue. The esthetic results are exceptional and appear to be durable.

Tongue Reconstruction

The most difficult of all problems faced by the maxillofacial surgeon in head and neck reconstruction is without question tongue reconstruction, because of the spectrum and complexity of the functions of the tongue. Disruption of normal visceral sensory mechanisms also disrupts the feedback required in the proper formation and propagation of a bolus to initiate swallowing. A complex interaction between the tongue, lips, cheeks, and jaws is required to simply masticate food. Any disruption of the sensory input from the tongue interferes with this process. The sensory input from the tongue is also required to trigger protective laryngeal reflexes and therefore prevent aspiration.

Muscular function of the tongue is dependent on both its extrinsic and the intrinsic muscles. The intrinsic muscles are perhaps the most important, existing in an interlacing network of fiber bundles. This arrangement gives the tongue the ability to alter its shape and position, a critical function in articulation.

Rehabilitation of patients requiring glossectomy necessitates an understanding of the limitations inherent in the available reconstruction techniques and the utility of adjunct procedures.[35] No currently available reconstruction can provide an exact replacement of all of the functions of the tongue. Techniques most applicable are those that do not limit the

function of the residual tongue. A freely mobile, thin, and pliable lining is provided by the radial forearm flap, which offers the best opportunity for near normal mobility of the residual tongue in the reconstruction of partial glossectomy defects.

Following total glossectomy, establishment of a stable platform that the patient can bring in contact with the palate provides the greatest likelihood for restoring oral swallowing function. In the process of the initiation of the pharyngeal phase of swallowing, significant interaction is required from the tongue base. This process is called the two-pump theory and is described by McConnel.[36] The tongue base pushes forward like a piston, propelling the food bolus as the first of the pump actions. A negative pressure is then created in the hypopharynx by anterior elevation of the larynx. Permanent anterosuperior suspension of the larynx to the mandible is a simple and especially useful adjunct technique that compensates for the inability of the reconstructed tongue base to elevate and push forward, opening the pharyngoesophageal segment. This technique should be considered in all cases of resection involving the tongue base. Urken et al[37] provide an excellent description of a systematic method for the evaluation and reconstruction of glossectomy defects. They offer a conceptualization of oral cavity reconstruction that is extremely helpful, especially as it relates to glossectomy defects.

Small, lateral defects of the anterior mobile tongue and the posterior tongue base can be primarily closed without significant loss of function. Whenever the resection extends onto the floor of the mouth or the lateral pharyngeal wall, reconstruction with a thin, pliable flap helps maintain mobility. The radial forearm free flap is particularly suited to such a condition. Near total glossectomy or total glossectomy requires a reconstruction with much different attributes. In particular, a fixed, rather than mobile, reconstruction is desirable. Likewise, a bulky flap is necessary to allow the patient to initiate a bolus. Adjunct techniques are definitely required in these reconstructions.

Partial glossectomy

Case study: Figure 8-3 shows reconstruction of a squamous cell carcinoma of the lateral tongue. Although the tongue cancer was small on the surface, deep invasion was evident by palpation. An elective neck dissection is warranted in the absence of palpable or radiographically demonstrable disease within the nodal drainage system. In this example the neck dissection revealed occult neck metastases. The major issues that are related to reconstruction of partial glossectomy defects are restoration of sensation, appropriate restoration of bulk, and preservation of mobility. A fasciocutaneous free radial forearm flap was selected for several reasons. The forearm flap is thin and pliable. It can be reinnervated, and the bulk of the flap is adjustable by increasing the fascial and subcutaneous component of the flap. By carefully addressing all of these issues, reconstruction of a partial glossectomy defect can be accomplished with a high degree of success. This patient returned to her original employment as a marketing consultant for a telephone company.

A fasciocutaneous flap with minimal thickness, the radial forearm flap, can also be reinnervated through the anastomosis of the median antebrachial cutaneous nerve to the lingual nerve. The advantage of such a reconstruction is mobility. Minimal contracture is associated with the free tissue transfer. The flap has an extremely robust blood supply, allowing significant freedom in designing flaps to match the complex three-dimensional contours of the tongue, floor of the mouth, and lateral pharynx.

The radial forearm flap was introduced by Yang et al[38] and subsequently reported by others[39] prior to being popularized by Soutar et al.[40,41] Both Urken et al[42] and Dubner and Heller[43] reported the utilization of the median antebrachial cutaneous nerve for the reinnervation of the radial forearm flap.

An excellent review of the recovery of sensory function in innervated radial forearm flaps following hemiglossectomy is provided by Santamaria et al,[44] who catalogs the sensory recovery of 28 patients and analyzes the impact of age, smoking history, size of the reconstructed defect, administration of postoperative radiation therapy, recipient nerve, and neurorrhaphy technique. Two blinded examiners performed standard neurologic testing (two-point discrimination, light touch sensation, pain perception, and hot and cold discrimination). The tip, dorsal aspect, ventral surface, and floor of the mouth were analyzed separately and compared to the intact native tongue. The authors concluded that predictable return of sensation approaching a near normal level could be anticipated whenever the median antebrachial cutaneous nerve underwent neurorrhaphy to the transected lingual nerve in an end-to-end fashion. Postoperative radiation therapy had a detrimental effect on the recovery of light touch and pain perception. Sensory reeducation is an extremely important factor in the process of return of sensation in these flaps.

Fig 8-3 (a) The palpable tongue cancer is outlined with hashed lines. An additional three-dimensional cuff of normal-appearing tissue must be resected because of the cancer's ability to invade adjacent tissue. (b,c) The depth of the lesion can be seen in the resection specimen. (d) Contraction of the tongue following resection gives a false indication of the size of the defect, which can only be accurately determined be stretching the tongue. (e) The antebrachial cutaneous nerve that supplies sensation to the volar forearm skin is seen in close proximity to the cephalic vein. (f) The harvested flap is seen, as well as two venous outflow tracts. The venae comitantes travel with the radial artery. The cephalic vein is seen separately. (g,h) Restoration of contour, bulk, and mobility are demonstrated.

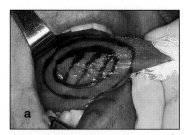

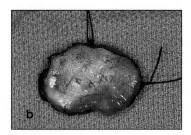

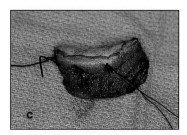

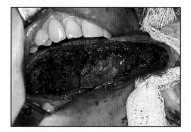

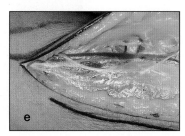

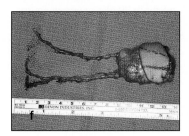

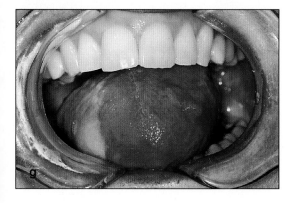

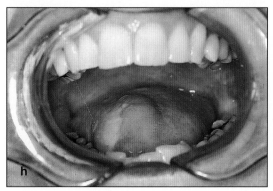

Near total or total glossectomy

Case study: Figure 8-4 shows a large squamous cell carcinoma of the tongue and tongue base that requires attention to a different set of issues than reconstruction of partial glossectomy defects. In such cases, bulk and sensation are much more important than mobility. The reconstructive surgeon must decide between restoration of bulk and restoration of sensation.

In this particular case, a rectus abdominus myocutaneous free flap allowed restoration of adequate bulk to initiate swallowing. Often such decisions are made based on the patient's motivation and whether or not the pulmonary status allows minimal aspiration during swallowing reeducation. This patient returned rapidly to an oral diet, his speech is easily understood, and he works full-time.

Fig 8-4 (a) A large squamous cell carcinoma of the tongue. The cancer involved over one half of the anterior mobile tongue and tongue base. (b) A rectus abdominus myocutaneous free flap is used for reconstruction. (c) The flap restores adequate bulk, allowing the patient to approximate the reconstruction to the palate, thereby forcing food and liquid into the pharynx to initiate reflexive swallowing. The patient eats orally. A percutaneous gastrotomy feeding tube was removed after radiation therapy.

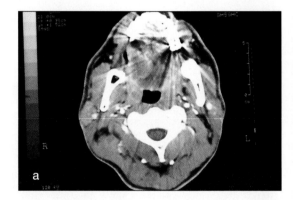

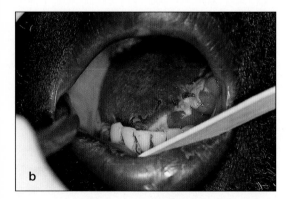

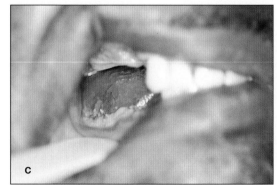

When volumes of the mobile tongue or the tongue base greater than one half of the normal tongue or bilateral hypoglossal nerve transection occur in the course of ablative head and neck surgery, the expected outcome is markedly diminished. Especially in the clinical setting of significant tongue base resection or sacrifice of both hypoglossal nerves, the main question often becomes whether or not a functioning larynx can be maintained because of concerns about the risk of aspiration. Several published reports have been dedicated to this problem.[35,45–47]

Salibian et al[45] described the outcome when using the osteomyocutaneous iliac flap 1 year following total or near total glossectomy in a group of eight survivors from an initial group of 12 patients. Six of the eight patients were able to take some form of food or liquid by mouth without aspiration. Weber et al[46] analyzed the results of a subgroup of 24 long-term survivors (greater than 2 years) of total or near total glossectomy with laryngeal preservation. Swallowing was initially achieved in 18 (67%); however, only 12 (44%) were able to maintain long-term deglutition. Urken[37] presents a scheme of patient analysis and reconstruction. Lyos et al[47] reported on the results of rectus abdominus free flap reconstruction in 14 patients who underwent resection of at least 75% of the tongue with preservation of the larynx. Twelve patients were successfully decannulated, and one interval laryngectomy was required. Fifty percent of the patients were able to take pureed food orally.

In the clinical setting of total or near total glossectomy, it is particularly critical to produce an appropriate volume of stable bulk tissue in the oral cavity. Upon closure of the mouth, this bulk should allow occlusion of the space within the oral cavity to propel a food bolus posteriorly.

Oral Lining Tissues

Case study: Figure 8-5 demonstrates an exophytic squamous cell carcinoma of the floor of the mouth in an edentulous patient. Resection necessitates marginal mandibulectomy. Restoration of the mandible, floor of the mouth, and ventral tongue lining was accomplished with a free radial forearm fasciocutaneous flap. Careful design of the skin portion of the flap allowed restoration of the complex three-dimensional site. The laxity designed into the reconstruction and the flexibility inherent in the radial forearm flap allowed mobility of the tongue without unseating the traditional mandibular complete denture. This finding was a surprise, since placement of implants was planned to improve denture retention. This patient wears his denture comfortably and has returned to the operation of the insurance company that he owns.

Reconstruction of the lining tissues of the oral cavity, particularly the floor of the mouth, lateral pharyngeal wall, and cheek, place specific requirements on the decisions of the reconstructive surgeon. Paramount among the characteristics of the flap selected are thinness, mobility, lack of contracture, and reliability. Donor site morbidity is an important secondary consideration. Following an appropriate preoperative evaluation, the reconstructive surgeon must develop a surgical plan based on the concept of the "reconstructive ladder," a useful intellectual exercise that requires assessment of the attributes and drawbacks of each available reconstruction method applicable to the ablative deformity. Defects of the oral cavity lining tissues may be reconstructed with myriad techniques, including split-thickness skin grafts, temporalis flaps, and free radial forearm flap.

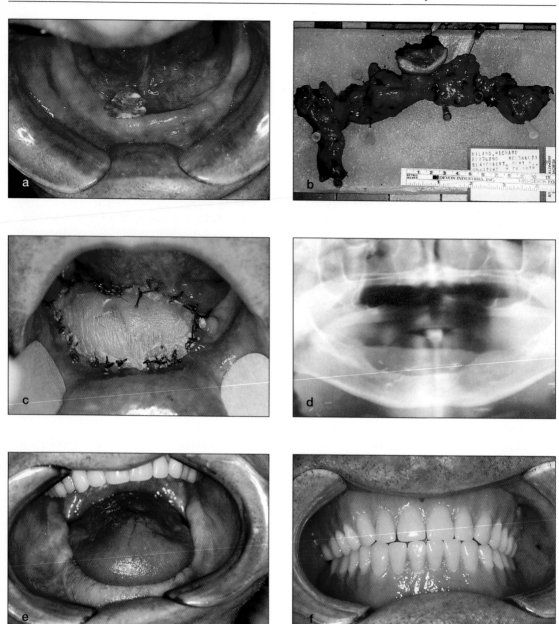

Fig 8-5 (a) Exophytic anterior floor of the mouth squamous cell carcinoma. (b) Resection of the lesion required marginal mandibulectomy and bilateral neck dissection. (c) The area was reconstructed with a free radial forearm fasciocutaneous flap. (d) The marginal mandibulectomy has compromised the denture-bearing area of the anterior mandible. (e,f) The flap provides flexibility of the tongue without tethering upon the tongue's movement, which would unseat a prosthesis. The complete denture is well tolerated. The patient was offered osseointegrated implants but declined. The prosthesis is stable.

Split-thickness skin grafting is applicable to only a small portion of oral cancer defects that result from the resection of very superficial tumors. The invasive nature of oral cavity cancers explains the rarity of this situation. Grafts are typically harvested from the anterolateral thigh. A medium thickness graft of 0.08 to 0.10 cm is preferred. The graft is inset to the stretched defect site to maximize the graft size and thereby decrease the overall effect of the contracture inevitable in the healing process. Direct adherence of the graft to the wound bed is required to allow the graft to "take." A bolster dressing is applied to ensure the direct apposition of the dermal side of the graft to the wound bed. The bolster prevents shearing forces from separating the graft and the formation of seroma or hematoma. The bolster is left in place for 1 week. The patient should take clear liquids by mouth until the bolster dressing is removed to prevent the accumulation of debris at the site of reconstruction. Survival of the graft is dependent upon diffusion for the first few days, after which time capillary ingrowth begins. Contracture of up to 50% is common with split-thickness skin grafting.

The temporalis muscle flap is extremely well suited to the reconstruction of defects of the lateral pharyngeal wall, soft palate, and cheek. Bradley and Brockbank[48] popularized the intraoral use of the temporalis flap. Continued interest in and support for the use of this flap has been exhibited by recent reports. Cheung[49] demonstrated the clinical implications of the vascular anatomy of the temporalis muscle and recommended an anatomically based technique for splitting the flap. He also demonstrated the rapid mucosalization of the temporalis muscle following oral transposition. Cordeiro and Wolfe[50] recently reported on the merits of the temporalis muscle flap and its application to clinical situations.

Summary

The surgical advances of the last decade offer the surgeon a number of improved reconstruction techniques in patients who have undergone resection of tumors of the head and neck. The ability of the reconstructive surgeon to conceptualize the three-dimensional characteristics of the defect is critical to the selection of the proper technique or combination of techniques. The reconstruction is tailored to the deformity in an attempt to achieve the best possible outcome. Sensory reinnervation, primary bony reconstruction, and osseointegration are particularly important characteristics of the modern head and neck reconstruction and contribute to the improvement in postoperative function and esthetics.

Early and continual interaction among the reconstructive surgeon, ablative surgeon, radiation oncologist, and chemotherapist is required to ensure that necessary interventions take place at the appropriate time. The establishment of a multidisciplinary conference in which all members of the team participate can meet this goal. Such an environment fosters close collaboration and significantly improves the quality of the patient evaluation, lessens the burden of interdisciplinary communication, and facilitates therapy. The multidisciplinary conference setting is also an extremely valuable teaching forum for residents. Patients can be presented prior to therapy and at intervals following treatment, as indicated by the clinical situation. This conference helps participants in the care of patients with head and neck cancer to understand the skills and developments within the other disciplines. When the ablative surgeon understands the limits and possibilities of modern head and neck reconstruction, better treatment decisions are made. Such collaboration has resulted in surgical resection being offered to patients who would otherwise have few therapeutic options.

Further development and refinement of head and neck reconstruction techniques will undoubtedly benefit patients with cancer. Subspecialization in reconstruction of the head and neck is now common. Such specialists have the best understanding of the requirements for reconstruction and can bring to bear the most current and useful advances.

References

1. Brown MR, McCullough TM, Funk GF, Graham SM, Hoffman HT. Resource utilization and patient morbidity in head and neck reconstruction. Laryngoscope 1997;107:1028.

2. Al Qattan MM, Boyd JB. Complications in head and neck microsurgery. Microsurgery 1993;14:187.

3. Singh B, Cordiero PG, Santamaria E, Shaha AE, Pfister DG, Shah JP. Factors associated with complications in microvascular reconstruction of head and neck defects. Plast Reconstr Surg 1999;103:403.

4. Kroll SS, Schusterman MA, Reece GP. Costs and complications in mandibular reconstruction. Ann Plast Surg 1992;29:341.

5. Carlson E, Marx R. Mandibular reconstruction using cancellous cellular bone grafts. Int J Oral Maxillofac Surg 1996;45:889.

6. Urken ML, Buchbinder D, Weinberg H, et al. Functional evaluation following microvascular oromandibular reconstruction of the oral cancer patient: A comparative study of reconstructed and nonreconstructed patients. Laryngoscope 1991;101:935.

7. Wagner JD, Coleman JJ, Weisenberger E. Predictive factors for functional recovery after free tissue transfer oromandibular reconstruction. Am J Surg 1998;176:430.

8. Komisar A, Warman S, Danziger E. A critical analysis of immediate and delayed mandibular reconstruction using A-O plates. Arch Otolaryngol Head Neck Surg 1989;115:830.

9. Komisar A. The functional result of mandibular reconstruction. Laryngoscope 1990;100:364.

10. Hidalgo D. Fibula free flap: A new method of mandible reconstruction. Plast Reconstr Surg 1989;84:71.

11. Sanders R, Mayou B. A new vascularized bone graft transferred by microvascular anastomosis as a free flap. Br J Surg 1979,66:787.

12. Taylor GI, Townsend P, Corlett R. Superiority of the deep circumflex iliac vessels as the supply for free groin flaps: Experimental work. Plast Reconstr Surg 1979;64:595.

13. Ramasastry SS, Granick MS, Futrell J. Clinical anatomy of the internal oblique muscle. J Reconstr Microsurg 1986;2:117.

14. Urken ML, Buchbinder D, Costantino PD, Sinha U, Okay D, Lawson W, Biller HF. Oromandibular reconstruction using microvascular composite flaps, report of 210 cases. Arch Otolaryngol Head Neck Surg 1998;124:46.

15. Shpitzer T, Neligan PC, Gullane PJ, et al. Oromandibular reconstruction with the fibular free flap, analysis of 50 consecutive flaps. Arch Otolaryngol Head Neck Surg 1997;123:939.

16. Wolff KD, Ervens J, Herzog K, Hoffmeister B. Experience with the osteocutaneous fibula flap: An analysis of consecutive reconstructions of composite mandibular defects. J Craniomaxillofac Surg 1996;24:330.

17. Lydiatt DD, Lydiatt WM, Hollins RR, Friedman A. Use of the free fibula flap in patients with prior failed mandibular reconstruction. Int J Oral Maxillofac Surg 1998;56:444.

18. Chang YM, Santamaria E, Wei FC, et al. Primary insertion of osseointegrated dental implants into fibula osteoseptocutaneous free flap for mandibular reconstruction. Plast Reconstr Surg 1998;102:680.

19. Urken ML, Weinberg H, Vickery C, Buchbinder D, Lawson W, Biller H. The internal oblique–iliac crest free flap in composite defects of the oral cavity involving bone, skin, and mucosa. Laryngoscope 1991;101:257.

20. Futran ND, Urken ML, Buchbinder D, Moscoso JF, Biller HF. Rigid fixation of vascularized bone grafts in mandibular reconstruction. Arch Otolaryngol Head Neck Surg 1995,121:70.

21. Ariyan S. The pectoralis major myocutaneous flap. A versatile flap for reconstruction in the head and neck. Plast Reconstr Surg 1979;63:73.

22. Marx RE, Smith BR. An improved technique for the development of the pectoralis major myocutaneous flap. Int J Oral Maxillofac Surg 1990;48:1168.

23. Moloy P, Gonzales F. Vascular anatomy of the pectoralis major myocutaneous flap. Arch Otolaryngol Head Neck Surg 1988,112:66.

24. Freeman JL, Walker EP, Wilson JSP, Shaw HJ. The vascular anatomy of the pectoralis major myocutaneous flap. Br J Plast Surg 1981;34:3.

25. Kiyokawa K, Tai Y, Tanabe HY, et al. A method that preserves circulation during preparation of the pectoralis major myocutaneous flap in head and neck reconstruction. Plast Reconstr Surg 1998;102:23–36.

26. Funk GF, Arcuri MR, Frodel JL. Functional dental rehabilitation of massive palatomaxillary defects: Cases requiring free tissue transfer and osseointegrated implants. Head Neck 1998;20:38.

27. Brown JS. Deep circumflex iliac artery free flap with internal oblique muscle as a new method of immediate reconstruction of the maxillectomy defect. Head Neck 1996;18:412.

28. Urken ML, Vickery C, Weinberg H, Buchbinder D, Lawson W, Biller HF. The internal oblique–iliac crest osseomyocutaneous free flap in oromandibular reconstruction: report of 20 cases. Arch Otolaryngol Head Neck Surg 1989;115:339.

29. Urken ML, Vickery C, Weinberg H, Buchbinder D, Biller HF. The internal oblique–iliac crest osseomyocutaneous microvascular free flap in head and neck reconstruction. J Reconstr Microsurg 1989;5:203.

30. Taylor G, Corlett RJ, Boyd B. The versatile deep inferior epigastric (inferior rectus abdominus) flap. Br J Plast Surg 1984;37:330.

31. Boyd JB, Taylor GI, Corlett R. The vascular territories of the superior epigastric and the deep inferior epigastric systems. Plast Reconstr Surg 1984;73:1.

32. Kyutoku S, Tsuji H, Inoue T, Kawakami K, Han F, Ogawa Y. Experience with the rectus abdominis myocutaneous flap with vascularized hard tissue for immediate orbitofacial reconstruction. Plast Reconstr Surg 1999;103:395.

33. Nakatsuka T, Harii K, Yamada A, Asato H, Ebihara S. Versatility of a free inferior rectus abdominus flap for head and neck reconstruction: Analysis of 200 cases. Plast Reconstr Surg 1994;93:762.

34. Urken ML, Turk JB, Weinberg H, Vickery C, Biller HF. The rectus abdominus free flap in head and neck reconstruction. Arch Otolaryngol Head Neck Surg 1991;117:857.

35. McConnel FM, Logeman JA, Rademaker AW. Surgical variables affecting postoperative swallowing efficacy in oral cancer patients: A pilot study. Laryngoscope 1994;104:87.

36. McConnel FM. Analysis of pressure generation and bolus transit during pharyngeal swallowing. Laryngoscope 1988;98:718.

37. Urken ML, Moscoso JF, Lawson W, Biller HF. A systematic approach to functional reconstruction of the oral cavity following partial and total glossectomy. Arch Otolaryngol Head Neck Surg 1994;120:589.

38. Yang G, Chen B, Gao Y, et al. Forearm free skin flap transplantation. Natl Med J China 1981,61:139.

39. Song R, Gao Y, Song Y, Yu Y, Song Y. The forearm flap. Clin Plast Surg 1982;9:21.

40. Soutar DS, Scheker LR, Tanner NSB, McGregor IA. The radial forearm flap: A versatile method for intraoral reconstruction. Br J Plast Surg 1983,36:1.

41. Soutar DS, McGregor IA. The radial forearm flap in intraoral reconstruction: The experience of 60 consecutive cases. Plast Reconstr Surg 1986;78:1.

42. Urken ML, Weinberg H, Vickery C, et al. The neurofasciocutaneous radial forearm flap in head and neck reconstruction: A preliminary report. Laryngoscope 1990;100:161.

43. Dubner S, Heller KS. Re-innervated radial forearm free flap in head and neck reconstruction. J Reconstr Microsurg 1992;8:467.

44. Santamaria E, Wei FC, Chen IH, Chuang DC. Sensation recovery on innervated radial forearm flap for hemiglossectomy reconstruction by using different recipient nerves. Plast Reconstr Surg 1999,103:450.

45. Salibian AH, Allison GR, Rappaport I, Krugman ME, McMicken BL, Etchepare TL. Total and subtotal glossectomy: Function after microvascular reconstruction. Plast Reconstr Surg 1990;85:513.

46. Weber RS, Ohlms L, Bowman J, Jacob R, Goepfert H. Functional results after total or near total glossectomy with laryngeal preservation. Arch Otolaryngol Head Neck Surg 1991;117:512.

47. Lyos AT, Evans GR, Perez D, Schusterman MA. Tongue reconstruction: Outcomes with the rectus abdominis flap. Plast Reconstr Surg 1999;103:442.

48. Bradley P, Brockbank J. The temporalis flap in oral reconstruction. A cadaveric, animal and clinical study. J Maxillofac Surg 1981;9:139.

49. Cheung LK. The vascular anatomy of the human temporalis muscle: Implications for surgical splitting techniques. Int J Oral Maxillofac Surg 1996;25:414.

50. Cordeiro PG, Wolfe SA. The temporalis muscle flap revisited on its centennial: Advantages, newer uses, and disadvantages. Plast Reconstr Surg 1996;98:980.

CHAPTER 9

Principles and Complications of Radiation Therapy

Mohan Suntharalingam, MD

Radiation therapy has a well-established role in the treatment of patients with carcinoma of the oral cavity. The therapeutic guidelines for its use have changed significantly over the past four decades as discoveries related to basic radiobiologic principles and the development of new technologies have paralleled improved understanding of the disease process. The basic principles of radiation involve the therapeutic application of high-energy X-rays that generate focal DNA damage within tumor cells.

In the 1940s, single modality therapy—either radical surgical resection or radiation alone—was the mainstay in the treatment of head and neck cancer. In part, the limitations of radiation therapy were defined by the prevailing concepts of the day which called for homogeneous doses delivered to large volumes of tissue. Total doses were based on the histologic appearance of the disease rather than the volume of tumor present. Radiation treatment was often reserved for recurrences after surgery, rather than being delivered in an adjuvant setting.

In the 1950s, basic radiobiologic principles were elucidated. These discoveries included the finding that the effect of radiation is dependent on the presence of oxygen, and the fact that the survival curve for irradiated cells revealed an exponential relationship between doses delivered and cell kill. These basic tenets led to the discovery of dose-response curves, which revealed that small increases in doses could lead to significant increases in tumor control. Perhaps equally important was the discovery that dose-response curves also reflected the sensitivity of normal tissue in the head and neck region.

During the 1960s, the first wave of the technology explosion included the widespread use of linear accelerators in many clinics. Sophisticated computer-based treatment planning systems were introduced for routine use in both external beam and brachytherapy dose-distribution calculations. Based on the complex anatomy of the head and neck region, computed tomography was introduced into radiation therapy clinics in the late 1970s in an attempt to improve the definition of target volumes and to identify surrounding normal tissues.

By the 1980s, this technology had developed to the point where three-dimensional reconstructions could be created from these two-dimensional images. These advances gave rise to the principles of conformal radiation therapy. The 1990s witnessed the second wave of major technologic innovation. The principle that has driven the development of conformal radiation therapy is based on the idea of maximizing dose-to-target volumes and minimizing the amount of radiation delivered to the surrounding normal tissue. The next step in the evolution of this technology has been the creation of intensity-modulated radiation therapy (IMRT), which delivers a spatially nonuniform radiation exposure from various points of reference that results in a homogeneous dose distribution at the target site.[1] The ability to deliver more conformal dose distributions and simultaneously spare normal tissue more effectively represents a significant advance in the development of radiation therapy.

External Beam Therapy

External beam radiation therapy has been used in both the definitive and adjuvant settings in patients with oral cavity carcinomas for many years. A basic understanding of the anatomy of this region revealed that each of the subsites within the oral cavity required an individual treatment approach. Treatment decisions account for the extent of the primary tumor and clinically involved lymph nodes, as well as the risk of occult, metastatic spread to the draining lymphatic nodal stations. The risk of microscopic spread helps to determine the extent of radiation therapy fields required to appropriately encompass all sites of potential disease. To develop a complete treatment plan, physicians must make appropriate therapy decisions regarding the treatment of the primary lesion as well as the neck lymph nodes.

The rate of lymph node metastasis is based on the location and extent of the primary tumor. A number of retrospective reviews have helped to determine the specific risk of lymph node involvement. Lindberg[2] reviewed the MD Anderson Cancer Center Registry and reported the incidence of clinically detectable lymph node involvement, based on stage, in patients presenting with squamous cell carcinoma of the head and neck. Byers[3] documented the incidence of microscopic lymph node involvement based on tumor stage when he published the cumulative pathologic results from neck dissection specimens obtained from patients with clinical stage N0 neck disease. Radiation administered to a clinically normal neck can achieve similar rates of local control compared to results with neck dissection, without disfigurement or functional deficits. This information helps to determine appropriate treatment requirements for patients based on the extent of the primary tumor. In general, therapeutic decisions regarding the treatment of the neck are made based on the mode of therapy used for the primary tumor. If the primary therapy is surgery, most patients undergo neck dissections. If radiation therapy is used initially, the nodes at risk are included within the radiation treatment fields.

Radiation therapy is commonly used following surgical resection when there is a significant risk of microscopic residual disease. Advantages of postoperative therapy include a reduced tumor burden and the availability of pathologic information to help determine the areas at greatest risk for harboring residual disease. Current indications for postoperative radiation therapy include close or positive margins, bone or cartilage involvement, extension of tumor into the soft tissues of the neck, perineural or vascular space invasion, extracapsular nodal extension, or multiple lymph node involvement. A retrospective analysis from the University of Florida revealed that primary tumors involving the oral cavity were associated with lower rates of control above the clavicles when compared to other head and neck sites.[4]

It has generally been considered standard practice to begin postoperative radiation therapy within 6 weeks of surgical resection. This recommendation is based on a retrospective analysis from the Memorial Sloan-Kettering Cancer Center which stated that prolongation of the interval between surgery and radiation for longer than 6 weeks was associated with an increased rate of failure.[5] An updated report from the same institution failed to confirm this finding. Other researchers have found no adverse effect with prolongation of this interval, as long as patients are able to complete therapy once they begin radiation treatment. The current recommendation is to initiate therapy as soon as the patient has healed sufficiently following surgery. This should typically be within 4 to 6 weeks; however, it may be necessary to wait longer, depending on the extent of resection.

Fletcher and colleagues[6] from the MD Anderson Cancer Center helped to set the standards of modern-day radiation therapy by establishing clinically effective doses for the management of head and neck malignancies. They clearly showed that 50 Gy delivered to a clinically normal neck could control microscopic disease in 95% of patients. Peters et al[7] reviewed the MD Anderson experience and reported that patients treated in the postoperative setting required a minimum dose of 57.6 Gy to the surgical bed to attain similar rates of local control. They theorized that the increased dose requirements were due to the changes in oxygenation status in the tissues that had been surgically manipulated. Their retrospective analysis also identified certain pathologic features that increased the risk of local regional failure. Specifically, they noted that positive surgical margins, multiple lymph nodes, and extracapsular nodal extension required doses of at least 63 Gy to optimize

regional control.[7] When radiation therapy is the definitive treatment for the primary tumor, doses are mainly determined by the size of the tumor and the fractionation schedule.

Altered Fractionation

Conventional radiation therapy fractionation schedules in the United States typically use doses between 1.8 and 2.0 Gy per day. Recently, a clearer understanding of the biologic relationship between time and dose has led to the investigation of altered fractionation therapy. A number of treatment schemes have been devised in an attempt to take advantage of the different radiation sensitivities of normal tissues and tumor. These schedules may also increase the number of tumor cells in the radiation-sensitive phase of the cell cycle during therapy. Increasing the total doses delivered to the tumor helps to counteract the effects of tumor cell proliferation that can occur during a typical course of external beam therapy. Clinical researchers have manipulated fraction size, overall treatment time, interfraction interval, and total dose in an attempt to improve cure rates for patients with head and neck carcinomas.

Hyperfractionation schedules are designed to decrease the dose per fraction while simultaneously increasing the number of fractions and the total dose. These schedules maintain similar overall treatment times (the number of days measured from the first day of treatment until the last) as compared to conventional therapy. This scheme aims to decrease late effects in comparison with acute effects, and to improve local tumor control with larger total doses. Accelerated fractionation schemes are defined by a decrease in overall treatment times while maintaining standard fraction sizes, number of fractions, and total dose. This allows for an increased tumor cell kill by avoiding the cellular repopulation that occurs with prolongation of overall treatment times. A combination of these two principles, known as *accelerated hyperfractionation,* attempts to increase tumor cell kill and to decrease the risk of long-term complications. Clinical experience with this particular regimen has led to the addition of a treatment break to allow for the recovery from the severe acute toxicities associated with this aggressive approach.

Three institutions in the United States have published their extensive experience with different altered fractionation schemes. The University of Florida used a true hyperfractionated regimen consisting of 1.2 Gy delivered twice a day (Monday through Friday), to a total dose of between 74.4 and 76.6 Gy. Massachusetts General Hospital reported its results with a split course, accelerated fractionation schedule. They used 1.6 Gy twice a day to deliver a total dose of 67.2 Gy in 6 weeks. This included a 10- to 14-day break after 38.4 Gy to allow for recovery from the normal tissue toxicities associated with this regimen. The MD Anderson Cancer Center developed a treatment regimen that is described as a concomitant boost technique. This scheme used a standard daily schedule of 1.8 Gy a day for a majority of the treatment period. The coned down boost is delivered as a second daily treatment during the final 2½ weeks of therapy with an additional 1.5 Gy per fraction given 4 to 6 hours after the morning treatment.

Each of these treatment schemes has shown improvements in local control rates as compared to standard fractionation schedules. Recently two randomized trials showed clear advantages to hyperfractionation schedules in the management of oropharyngeal cancer. To try and define the optimum total dose to be used with these twice-a-day schedules, the Radiation Therapy Oncology Group (RTOG) has completed a dose escalation study. This study included patients with advanced squamous cell carcinomas of the head and neck. The five-arm study examined dose levels between 67.2 and 81.6 Gy. An analysis of the data has shown that local control was best with doses between 72 and 76 Gy.[8] Recently the RTOG completed a four-arm, randomized study that included a standard daily treatment schedule and each of the three altered fractionation schemes previously outlined. The study attempted to determine which of these schedules would result in the best local control and survival rates in patients with squamous cell carcinoma of the head and neck. It has now closed and the results are pending.

Brachytherapy

The routine use of primary radiation therapy in patients with oral cavity carcinomas is often complicated by the increased risks of normal tissue toxicities associated with delivery of therapy in this anatomic region. Standard daily external radiation therapy for early stage lesions produces similar cure rates compared to surgical resection; however, the risk of soft tissue and bone necrosis is substantially higher than that in other head and neck subsites. To overcome the limitations of external photon beam therapy, many researchers have studied the addition of brachytherapy or intraoral cone irradiation in appropriately selected patients.

Brachytherapy refers to the use of radioactive isotopes to deliver localized doses of radiation that can treat tumor-bearing areas while simultaneously sparing surrounding normal tissues. Investigators at MD Anderson and the University of Florida have shown that the application of interstitial radioactive implants can achieve excellent rates of local control and cure in early stage lesions without the associated risks of normal tissue damage.[9] These institutions used radium needles as temporary implants that were placed within a prefabricated mold and then inserted directly into regions such as the floor of the mouth. Through the years other isotopes, such as iridium 192 and cesium 137, have gained popularity because of the advantages they offer in terms of radiation safety. These lower energy isotopes require less shielding, and they afford the opportunity to use afterloading techniques. These advances allow physicians to place afterloading catheters in the tumor bed while the patient is in the operating room. Pretreatment dosimetry verifies that adequate doses of radiation will be delivered to all tissues deemed to be at risk for harboring cancerous cells prior to the implantation of the radiation sources. The radioactive sources may be loaded into position within the catheters once the patient has been returned to the hospital room and the appropriate shielding is in place. This results in a significant decrease in radiation exposure to hospital personnel.

Brachytherapy allows for the precise delivery of localized therapy with continuous low-dose irradiation. The biologic effect of this therapy may be equated to an infinite number of small doses of external radiation therapy that can deliver a tumoricidal dose within a short overall treatment time. Very early lesions in the floor of the mouth or the tongue may be amenable to brachytherapy alone, but most early stage lesions require combination therapy to cover all potential sites of disease. When prescribing doses with brachytherapy, consideration must be given to the rate at which the radiation is delivered. Most implants in the head and neck region require a volumetric analysis of dose deposition. Typically, most

implants are constructed to deliver between 40 and 55 Gy per hour at a predetermined position within the volume. Sophisticated treatment planning computers are now available to help calculate the doses delivered throughout the entire treatment volume. It is not unusual to see a significantly higher dose of radiation in the center of the implant as compared to the regions located on the periphery.

Intraoral Cone Irradiation

Intraoral cone irradiation has also been used in an attempt to safely deliver adequate doses of radiation to the oral cavity. A radiation delivery device focuses a superficially penetrating radiation beam on a small volume of diseased tissue, while sparing adjacent normal structures. Clinical investigators have reported excellent control rates for early lesions located on the alveolar ridge, tongue, and floor of the mouth regions. Wang and Biggs[10] at Massachusetts General Hospital have reported their long-term experience with intraoral cone therapy and convincingly shown that it is both safe and efficacious in appropriately selected patients. Patients must be edentulous to receive this treatment, and precise placement of the cone on top of the lesion is mandatory to ensure accurate radiation delivery. A tumor must be located in a region far enough away from the mandible, and anterior enough within the oral cavity, to allow for the placement of the cone on a daily basis. Daily fractions of 2.5 to 3 Gy are commonly used for total boost doses of between 15 and 21 Gy.

Most patients are treated with a combination of intraoral cone therapy followed by external beam radiation. It is sequenced in this manner to account for the expected mucositis associated with external beam therapy, which might limit a patient's ability to tolerate daily cone placement, as well as to provide the best evaluation of true tumor extent prior to any treatment. Intraoral cone therapy can now be delivered with either orthovoltage or electron beam therapy. Both types of radiation are considered superficially penetrating, so there are limits to the type of tumors that can be treated effectively. Lesions greater than 1 cm thick may be underdosed at their deep margins because of the rapid falloff of dose associated with these types of radiation. The cones themselves often limit the application of this technology due to the patient's inability to accommodate the bulky device within the oral cavity. Patients who have tumors of the anterior tongue must have adequate mobility to allow for the accurate placement of the cone on a daily basis. Floor of the mouth tumors are often best suited for this therapy which, compared to interstitial brachytherapy, can achieve equal rates of local control with lower rates of osteoradionecrosis of the mandible.

Treatment Philosophies

Carcinoma of the lip

Cancers of the lip usually arise on the mucosa of the lower lip or the vermilion border as a result of chronic sun exposure. Decisions regarding treatment are typically made based on location and size of the primary tumor. While surgery can be used for early lesions, the location of the tumor may lead to significant functional and esthetic deficits. Primary radiation therapy is typically used for any lesion that would require resection of the commissure. External electron beam therapy

or an interstitial implant is expected to offer a 90% chance of cure in early stage lesions. As the size of the tumor increases, radiation therapy is typically offered as the primary treatment modality. These cases require prophylactic treatment of the draining lymphatics in the submental and submandibular regions, as well as adequate margins around the primary tumor. External beam therapy is often used with doses of 3 Gy per fraction to total doses of between 30 and 50 Gy followed by implant. Multiple institutional reports have shown local control rates between 75% and 85% for lesions greater than 2 cm.[11]

Anterior two thirds of the tongue

Most patients presenting with early stage cancers of the tongue are offered either surgery or definitive radiation therapy that combines external beam therapy and interstitial implants. Either of these therapies can achieve cure in 85% to 90% of early stage lesions; however, if radiation therapy is chosen, a combination of therapies must be used. Researchers from both MD Anderson and the University of Florida have shown a direct relationship between the amount of therapy delivered with brachytherapy and improved local control rates in tumors treated with implant therapy plus external beam therapy.[12] In fact, external beam therapy alone has led to inferior results and higher rates of normal tissue toxicities when compared to surgical resection. The primary lymph node drainage includes the submandibular and anterior cervical nodal chains. Patients must either undergo an elective neck dissection or prophylactic neck irradiation, depending on how the primary tumor is managed. Locally advanced lesions are typically treated with surgery followed by postoperative radiation therapy.

Floor of the mouth

Tumors in the floor of the mouth are often treated in the same manner as those found in the anterior tongue. Definitive radiation therapy includes a combination of external beam therapy and brachytherapy to maximize local control with early stage lesions. Intraoral cone therapy is often used instead of interstitial implants, depending on the anatomy of this region. In fact, surgery is usually chosen because of the similar rates of control and the significant risk of bone and soft tissue damage associated with radiation therapy in this area. T3 and T4 lesions require primary surgical resection followed by adjuvant radiation therapy based on pathologic findings. This approach leads to the best chance for both local control and survival. Patients who present with surgically unresectable disease are offered enrollment in institutional studies that combine radiation therapy with concurrent chemotherapy. These therapies may be given as definitive management or as induction treatment that attempts to downstage the tumor and render it amenable to surgical resection.

Buccal mucosa

Small lesions involving the oral commissure are best treated with radiation therapy to obtain the optimal functional outcome. Radiation fields encompass the primary tumor plus the first echelon of draining lymph nodes in the ipsilateral neck. If the tumor extends into the gingivobuccal sulcus or onto the adjacent gingiva, external beam therapy is absolutely required. Retrospective studies have revealed that tumors in this region have an increased rate of marginal failures, so increased field sizes must be used as part of the initial treatment. Studies dating back to

the 1960s have shown local control rates from 60% to 90% with radiation, depending on the size of the primary lesion.[13] Many lesions are not amenable to primary radiation therapy because of their proximity to the underlying bone. Patients who have been treated with surgical resection have achieved a 5-year survival rate of 80%.

Retromolar trigone

This anatomic region is sometimes included with tumors of the anterior tonsillar pillar; however, lesions in this area behave similar to those in the lower gingiva. This region is defined as the small triangular surface covering the ascending ramus behind the third molar. Tumors here are most commonly treated with surgical resection because of the significant morbidity associated with high-dose radiation in this area. Invasion of the periosteum occurs early in the disease process; however, cortex involvement is rare due to the dense bone in this region. If radiation therapy is used for early stage lesions, intraoral cone therapy is typically part of the treatment plan used to safely deliver adequate doses. Locally advanced tumors are managed with a combination of surgery and postoperative radiation.

Normal Tissue Toxicities

The effects of radiation therapy are usually divided into acute effects (those experienced either during or shortly after the completion of treatment) and late effects (those manifested months to years after therapy). Acute effects are most often self-limited; however, they can severely limit a patient's ability to complete therapy as originally prescribed.

Late effects tend to be chronic and progressive because they are a consequence of injury to slowly proliferating or nonproliferating tissues. The development of moderate or severe acute effects does not directly predict the risk of late effects, as these two types of injury are typically a result of disassociated processes. Attempts to reduce the frequency of either type of normal tissue injury must be rooted in the basic biologic concepts of normal tissue repair of sublethal damage, reassortment of cells within the sensitive portions of the cell cycle, repopulation, and reoxygenation. These radiobiologic discoveries have formed the basis for conventional, fractionated radiation therapy. Dividing a dose of radiation into fractions spares normal tissue because of the ability of the cells to repair sublethal damage between subsequent doses.

The two most important determinants of acute toxicities are the dose given per fraction and the overall treatment time. Larger doses given as daily fractions can lead to an increased risk of acute side effects, whereas prolongation of overall treatment time leads to a significant sparing effect. The risk of developing most late toxicities is primarily a function of the amount of radiation delivered with each fraction, the time between fractions, and the total dose received.

As the mechanisms of normal tissue cell injury have been elucidated, it has become apparent that the potential complications must be considered as total doses of radiation are pushed higher, and therapies should be combined in an attempt to improve cure rates. The oral cavity contains many structures that are acutely sensitive to radiation therapy, including mucous membranes, skin, facial hair, salivary tissue, and taste buds. Tissues that are at risk for late morbidity include soft tissue, muscle, salivary glands, bone, thyroid, and spinal cord.

Mucous membranes

The mucous membranes that cover the oral cavity are among the most radiation-sensitive tissue systems in the body. Mild erythema develops within the first week during a conventional course of 1.8 to 2.0 Gy per day. By the end of the second week, this reddened mucosal membrane develops small white patches called *mucositis* (or false membrane formation). These areas are dead surface epithelium with an inflammatory infiltrate seen on a moist background. At this point, most patients typically report the onset of a sore throat and difficulty swallowing. As therapy continues, these patchy areas become confluent by the third or fourth week. The lateral borders of the tongue and buccal mucosa are the most commonly involved sites, whereas regions such as the hard palate, gingival ridges, and dorsum of the tongue tend to be spared. Patients who have metal-based dental restorations are at increased risk of developing brisk mucositis on the adjacent buccal mucosa and tongue secondary to scattered low-energy electrons created by the photon interaction with the metal. Typically, the surrounding tissues can be spared by increasing the distance between the crowns and mucosal surface with simply designed tissue spacers.

Coutard[14] described an interesting phenomenon known as *tumoritis* that has historically aided radiation oncologists in precise tumor definition. He noted that mucositis typically first appears over the tumor itself during the first 5 to 7 days. Previously undetected areas of adjacent tumor spread can help to define appropriate boost fields for the final cone down of radiation therapy. Weekly examinations of patients undergoing radiation therapy is vital to confirm adequate treatment field coverage, as well as to provide clinical evidence of acceptable dose delivery.

During a standard 7-week course of therapy that encompasses the oral cavity, a patient is routinely instructed to use a number of mouth-rinses to palliate the symptoms associated with mucositis. Salt and soda solutions are typically prescribed during the first few weeks to maintain appropriate oral hygiene. As treatment continues, a broad spectrum antimicrobial agent such as chlorhexidine is used in an attempt to reduce the severity of mucositis.[15] This substance is bound to the mucosal surfaces after each use (usually given as 15 mL swish and expectorate four times a day) and is effective against both bacteria and fungal infections. Opioid analgesics may become necessary after a few weeks of treatment to manage the pain associated with mucosal irritation and to prevent further nutritional compromise. One month after the completion of therapy, mucositis resolves in 90% of patients.

Sense of taste

Approximately 1 week into therapy, most patients report an alteration in their sense of taste. This is a direct result of the radiation's effect on taste buds, which are located throughout the oral cavity and found abundantly on the circumvallate papillae. They are also found scattered throughout the fungiform papillae located in the anterior two thirds of the tongue, and along the posterolateral surfaces of the tongue. The four primary taste sensations are controlled by different locations on the tongue. For example, the anterior tongue and tip control sweet tastes, and the lateral sides control sour. Bitter tastes are picked up by the circumvallate papillae, and salty tastes can be detected throughout the tongue.

By the time 20 to 40 Gy have been received, patients report a significant increase in the degree of loss of taste. Patients who possess a higher level of pretreatment taste acuity often suffer a more rapid sense of loss during therapy. It has been suggested that loss of taste is due to damage to the microvilli of the taste cells.[16] At the completion of therapy, acuity of taste is recovered first and then most patients report slow recovery of various taste sensations over the next 1 to 2 months. While many patients have no subjective complaints of taste loss, many have measurable losses of both bitter and salty sensations. It is rare for patients to experience long-term deficits; however, a portion of this subjective loss can result from xerostomia, which does affect taste acuity. A few uncontrolled studies have suggested that zinc therapy after completion of therapy may alleviate symptoms of patients whose sense of taste does not return to normal.

Salivary tissue

The major salivary glands, including the parotid, submandibular, and sublingual glands, produce 70% to 80% of the salivary flow. Minor salivary glands located throughout the oral cavity produce the remaining 20% to 30%. Under normal conditions, the submandibular glands, which consist of both mucous and serous acini, have the ability to produce as much saliva as the parotids (consisting entirely of serous acini), whereas the sublingual glands (mucous secretors) typically generate only 2% to 5% of the total salivary volume.[17] When stimulation occurs, the parotid glands dominate production. If a patient's treatment fields encompass both submandibular and sublingual glands but spare a significant portion of the parotid glands, it is possible that few subjective changes will be noted. The degree of xerostomia induced by radiation therapy is directly related to the location and amount of salivary tissue in the treatment field.

Most patients receiving conventional external beam therapy that encompasses the paired major salivary glands report a subjective change after only a few treatments. Some investigators have reported up to a 50% decrease in salivary production after the first week of therapy.[18] The subsequent decline is less dramatic, but continual. Radiation to the salivary glands has the direct effect of decreased production, and as a result an increase in salivary sodium concentration, a decrease in pH level, and a subsequent rise in oral yeast flora can occur. The consistency of the saliva changes dramatically during the course of therapy. Patients often complain of great difficulty handling their secretions after radiation therapy because their saliva has become thick and ropy. This occurs as a direct result of intrinsic radiation sensitivity of the serous acini located within the parotid glands. The saliva that is produced from these glands after radiation therapy is tenacious as a result of a disproportionate amount of mucinous acini activity and serous acini atrophy.

Recently, an increasing body of data has emerged that suggests a possible benefit to the use of pilocarpine to decrease the severity of postradiation xerostomia. Initially, researchers explored the role of this agent in the management of radiation-induced salivary gland dysfunction. Multiple studies revealed objective improvements in salivary flow with the use of pilocarpine following radiation. Unfortunately, many patients did not report subjective improvements in oral moisture, which led to an examination of the role of prophylactic pilocarpine in the prevention of xerostomia by administering the drug during the course of radiation therapy. Researchers at Wayne State University reported an early experience with the drug given concurrently with daily radiation that revealed a significant improvement in salivary production. Patients' subjective assessment of oral mucosal changes reflected improvements in oral dryness and pain associated with mucositis.[19] A randomized national clinical trial is currently seeking to validate this initial experience, which suggests a significant benefit to the use of pilocarpine.

Patients must have a clear understanding of the potential salivary changes that radiation therapy may cause and an effective strategy for dealing with them. These significant lifestyle changes must be addressed at the time of initial consultation. Patients are routinely given a wide variety of instructions in an attempt to decrease the symptoms associated with the chronic changes seen with decreased salivary production. These instructions include avoidance of alcohol-based mouthrinses, frequent sips of water with lemon drops, special food preparation, avoidance of food containing a high percentage of sugar and alcohol, and the use of artificial saliva solutions.

Osteoradionecrosis

During a typical course of radiation therapy for oral cavity malignancies, a significant portion of bone is usually included within the treatment fields. High-dose radiation carries a risk of ischemia and fibrosis to the mandible and maxilla, which can lead to avascular necrosis, sequestration, pathologic fractures, and secondary infections. Microscopically, these changes are characterized by damage to the cellular elements, which results in an inflammatory infiltrate and obvious vascular changes. Most cases of osteoradionecrosis (ORN) result from damage to tissues overlying the bone as opposed to direct damage to the bone itself. Typically, soft tissue necrosis of the gingival mucosa and bone exposure occurs prior to the development of ORN. The gingiva of the mandible is more susceptible to the effects of radiation than is that of the maxilla.

The most common sites of ORN are the mandibular arch and the mylohyoid ridge.

Several risk factors, including amount of bone in treatment ports, total doses, smoking, and subsequent trauma, have been identified.[20] Patients who have undergone radiation therapy and subsequently undergo dental extractions are at high risk for the development of ORN. The microvascular changes that occur within the bone are permanent, and therefore the risk of ORN remains throughout a patient's lifetime. In fact, ORN often occurs many years after the completion of therapy.

Effective strategies have been constructed to decrease the risk of radiation-induced bone damage. Preventive measures have included careful pretreatment, dental evaluations, and extraction of all grossly diseased teeth prior to treatment. In addition, primary closure of the mucosa, prophylaxis with broad spectrum antibiotics, and adequate healing intervals prior to therapy all help to decrease the risk of ORN development. Most importantly, dental personnel caring for these patients must have a clear understanding of the precise radiation therapy ports each patient will receive.

Once therapy has begun, extractions should be avoided. If it becomes necessary to remove a tooth, hyperbaric oxygen should be considered for any surgery involving bone that has received 50 Gy or more.[21] Randomized studies document the ability of hyperbaric oxygen to decrease the incidence and severity of radiation-associated bone necrosis following dental extractions. A typical hyperbaric oxygen schedule might include 20 consecutive 90-minute dives at 2.4 to 2.6 atmospheres. If ORN occurs, aggressive intervention can often limit the long-term sequelae. Local irrigation, topical enzyme solutions, and antibiotics are followed by surgical debridement as needed. Hyperbaric oxygen is often used both before and after surgical intervention.

Skin

The epidermis consists mostly of stratified squamous epithelium and a deeper basal layer. The basal layer contains mitotically active cells that continuously replace the keratinized cellular layers that are exfoliated. In the past, standard radiation therapy practices using orthovoltage treatment machines placed high doses of radiation in the skin and subcutaneous tissues. This resulted in excessive toxicity and limited practitioners' ability to deliver adequate radiation therapy doses. Today's megavoltage technology uses penetrating, high-energy beams that allow for appropriate dose delivery to midline structures when treating with opposed photon beams, with a simultaneous ability to spare the superficial tissues.

During a standard continuous course of radiation therapy, a patient often experiences acute skin toxicities such as erythema, peeling, and hyperpigmentation. The peeling that is seen results from a direct effect on the basal layer where mitotically active cells are killed. Patients often report an increased sensitivity to touch and persistent itching during this time. In cases of severe skin reactions, moist desquamation can occur when the basal cell layer's ability to repopulate has been overcome by increased cell death. These lesions heal spontaneously in 2 to 4 weeks, with little risk of long-term damage.

Summary

Carcinomas of the oral cavity continue to represent a significant therapeutic challenge. Cancer specialists who treat these patients must have a clear understanding of the anatomic relationships of this region as well as the patterns of tumor spread. Radiation therapy will continue to have a major role in the management of early stage disease, as technologic advances have improved the ability to maximize doses to well-defined targets while simultaneously limiting radiation doses to the surrounding normal tissue. Future research will focus on the application of these innovations within a multidisciplinary treatment scheme. It is clear that the reduction of treatment-related toxicities will continue to be emphasized in early stage tumors. It is equally clear that the successful combination of surgery, radiation therapy, and chemotherapy will be required to significantly improve the cure rates for those patients with locally advanced disease.

References

1. Purdy JA. The development of intensity modulated radiation therapy. In: Sternick E (ed). The Theory and Practice of Intensity Modulated Radiation Therapy, 1997:8.

2. Lindberg RD. Distribution of cervical lymph node metastases from squamous cell carcinoma of the upper respiratory and digestive tracts. Cancer 1972;29: 1446–1449.

3. Byers RM. Modified neck dissection: A study of 967 cases from 1970 to 1980. Am J Surg 1985;150: 414–421.

4. Amdur RJ, et al. Postoperative radiation for squamous cell carcinoma of the head and neck: An analysis of treatment results and complications. Int J Radiat Oncol Biol Phys 1989;16:25–36.

5. Vikram B. Importance of time interval between surgery and postoperative radiation therapy in combined management of head and neck cancer. Int J Radiat Oncol Biol Phys 1979;5:1837–1840.

6. Fletcher GH. Lucy Wortham lecture: Subclinical disease. Cancer 1984;53:1274–1284.

7. Peters LJ, Goepfert H, Ang, KK, et al. Evaluation of the dose for postoperative radiation therapy of head and neck cancer: First report of a prospective randomized trial. Int J Radiat Oncol Biol Phys 1993;26:3–11.

8. Cox JD. Dose response for local control with hyperfractionated radiation therapy in advanced carcinoma of the upper aerodigestive tracts. Int J Radiat Oncol Biol Phys 1990;18:515–521.

9. Ellingwood KE, Million RR, Mitchell TP. A preloaded radium needle implant device for maintenance of needle spacing. Cancer 1981;496–502.

10. Wang CC, Biggs PJ. Technical and radiotherapeutic considerations of intraoral cone electron beam radiation therapy for head and neck cancer. Semin Radiat Oncol 1992;2:171–179.

11. Million RR, Cassisi NJ, Mancuso AA. Oral cavity. In: Million RR, Cassisi NJ (eds). Management of Head and Neck Cancer: A Multidisciplinary Approach, ed 2. Philadelphia: Lippincott, 1994.

12. Mendenhall WM, Van Cise WS, Bova FJ, et al. Analysis of time-dose factors in squamous cell carcinoma of the oral tongue and floor of mouth treated with radiotherapy. Int J Radiat Oncol Biol Phys 1981;7:1005–1011.

13. MacComb WS, Fletcher GH, Healy JE. Intraoral cavity. In: MacComb WS, Fletcher GH (eds). Cancer of the Head and Neck. Baltimore: Williams & Wilkins, 1967:89–151.

14. Coutard H. Roentgen therapy of epitheliomas of the tonsillar region, hypopharynx and larynx from 1920–1926. Am J Roentgenol Radium Ther 1932;28: 313–331.

15. Ferretti GA, Hansen IA, Whittenburg K, et al. Therapeutic use of chlorhexidine in bone marrow transplant patients: Case studies. Oral Surg Oral Med Oral Pathol 1987;63:683–687.

16. Conger AD. Loss and recovery of taste acuity in patients irradiated in the oral cavity. Radiat Res 1973; 53:338–347.

17. Enfors B. The parotid and submandibular secretion in man: Quantitative recordings of the normal and pathological activity. Acta Otolaryngol 1962;172(suppl): 1–67.

18. Makkonen TA, Edelman L, Forsten L. Salivary flow and caries prevention in patients receiving radiotherapy. Proc Finn Dent Soc 1986;82:93–100.

19. LeVeque FG, Fontanesi J, Klein BJ, et al. Pilot study to determine if oral pilocarpine given concurrently with head and neck irradiation can decrease the incidence and severity of salivary gland dysfunction [abstract]. Proc Am Soc Clin Oncol 1996;15:516.

20. Parsons JT, Fitzgerald CR, Hood CI, et al. A re-evaluation of split course technique for squamous cell carcinoma of the head and neck. Int J Radiat Oncol Biol Phys 1980;6:1645–1652.

21. Marx RE, Johnson RP, Kline SN. Prevention of osteoradionecrosis: A randomized prospective clinical trial of hyperbaric oxygen versus penicillin. J Am Dent Assoc 1985;111:49–54.

CHAPTER 10

Principles and Complications of Chemotherapy

Barbara A. Conley, MD

Chemotherapy for Cancers of the Head and Neck

In the past several years, the use of chemotherapy has increased in frequency in the treatment of patients with squamous cell carcinoma of the head and neck. Combinations of chemotherapeutic agents as well as combinations of chemotherapy with radiation and/or surgery are common. Chemotherapy can be used either with the primary modality of treatment (eg, surgery and/or radiation therapy), prior to the primary modality (neoadjuvant), after the primary modality in patients who have been rendered free of gross tumor (adjuvant), or palliatively for recurrent or metastatic disease.

Chemotherapy administration

Generally, patients must meet certain criteria to be considered candidates for treatment with chemotherapy. Performance status is an important predictor of prognosis. Patients who are able to function relatively normally and who spend at least 50% of their time out of bed tolerate chemotherapy better and are more likely to respond to treatment than patients who spend most of their day in bed. Patients must also be reliable for follow-up to be candidates for chemotherapy, because toxicities from chemotherapy administration can be severe and can occur from 1 to 3 weeks after the chemotherapy administration. Good liver, kidney, and bone marrow function is also required to avoid severe, permanent function loss.

The route and schedule of chemotherapy administration depends on the particular agent being used. Some regimens require that chemotherapeutic drugs be given in a certain sequence. Common regimens include continuous intravenous infusions for 3 to 5 days (eg, 5-fluorouracil, possibly taxanes), short infusion or bolus intravenous administration every 3 to 4 weeks, and weekly administration by intravenous bolus or short infusion.

Several chemotherapeutic agents have shown activity in squamous cell carcinoma of the head and neck. These agents are usually identified in phase II treatment trials, in which up to 40 patients with head and neck cancer receive the single agent. The number of complete responses (eg, complete disappearance of tumor for at least 4 weeks) and partial responses (eg, at least 50% decrease in the sum of the products of the perpendicular diameters of all tumors) comprise the response rate. Sometimes minimal responses (25% to 50% decrease in the sum of the products of the perpendicular diameters of all tumors) are included in the response rate as well. Responses to single chemotherapy agents rarely last more than 3 months, despite continued treatment with the agent. The response rate decreases with use of subsequent agents.

Although several chemotherapeutic agents have shown response rates of 15% to 25% in squamous cell carcinoma of the head and neck, only a few of these agents are used commonly.

Cisplatin is probably the single most common agent in use for head and neck cancer. It is usually given as a short intravenous infusion every 3 to 4 weeks and has a response rate as a single agent of 30% to 40%. Cisplatin is thought to cause cell death by causing intrastrand DNA crosslinks. Toxic side effects include renal damage, which can be prevented with aggressive hydration and diuresis during administration, high-frequency hearing loss, moderate myelosuppression about 2 weeks after administration, moderate hair loss, neurotoxicity (tingling and numbness of fingers and toes), and allergic reactions. It can also cause severe and prolonged nausea and vomiting, which may increase renal damage because of dehydration. Cisplatin may cause severe hypomagnesemia and hyponatremia; serum electrolyte levels need to be followed in patients throughout treatment. Administration of cisplatin has become easier over the past several years because of the development of newer, more powerful antiemetic agents.

Carboplatin is another platinum-containing chemotherapy drug that can be used in the treatment of squamous cell carcinoma of the head and neck. The mechanism of action of carboplatin is similar to that of cisplatin. Carboplatin can be administered as an intravenous bolus every 3 to 4 weeks, in place of cisplatin for patients with moderate renal dysfunction. Carboplatin administration is not associated with severe renal damage such as that encountered with cisplatin, but is associated with a greater degree of myelosuppression, particularly thrombocytopenia. The dose of carboplatin can be targeted to achieve a specified exposure and calculated using the patient's creatinine clearance, so that a uniform area under the plasma concentration time curve (AUC) can be approached for any patient, even those with compromised renal function.[1] Cisplatin (or carboplatin) can be combined with other chemotherapeutic agents, either in full doses or in small doses that may enhance the effects of concurrent radiation therapy. Two classes of agents with which the platinum chemotherapy agents are commonly combined are 5-fluorouracil and taxanes.

5-Fluorouracil (5FU) is usually given with cisplatin. Generally, cisplatin (100 mg/m^2 body surface area) is given on day 1, followed by a 4- to 5-day continuous infusion of 5FU at a dose of 1 g/m^2 per 24 hours. 5-Fluorouracil inhibits thymidylate synthase, an enzyme necessary for DNA synthesis, and can inhibit RNA synthesis as well. The toxicities of 5FU depend on the schedule of administration. Continuous infusion schedules can be associated with severe mucositis, diarrhea, decreased white blood cell count, hair loss, skin discoloration, and hand-foot syndrome, a desquamative condition affecting the palms and soles. Rarely, cardiac and central nervous system toxicity can be seen. Bolus administration schedules are more commonly associated with myelosuppression, but can be complicated by diarrhea and mucositis as well. An individual patient's tolerance of a 5-day infusion of 5FU as previously described is variable, and the infusion can be stopped at the first sign of mucositis (usually manifested as a tingling sensation) to prevent more severe mucositis. 5-Fluorouracil has also been given with radiation therapy and is considered a radiation sensitizer. Mucositis is expected to be more severe with 5FU plus radiation than with radiation alone.

The taxanes are a relatively new class of compounds that have activity in several solid tumors, including squamous cell carcinoma of the head and neck. The mechanism of action of these agents is stabilization of microtubules. This stabilization inhibits dissolution of the mitotic spindle, which leads to cell death. The two currently available drugs in this class are paclitaxel and docetaxel. The taxanes are usually given as a short (1- to 3-hour) intravenous infusion every 3 to 4 weeks, although paclitaxel has been administered weekly either as a radiation sensitizer or in larger doses[2,3] and has been administered as continuous infusions either with other chemotherapeutic agents or with radiation therapy.[4]

The most common toxicities of paclitaxel are myelosuppression and neurotoxicity. Myelosuppression can be severe, and nadirs can occur between 1 and 2 weeks after drug administration. Paclitaxel is insoluble in water and must be administered in a mixture of Cremophor and ethanol. Allergic reactions can occur during or shortly after the paclitaxel infusion and are thought to be related to the diluent. Therefore, paclitaxel administration is preceded by premedication consisting of H_2 receptor blockers, steroids, and diphenhydramine.

The most common toxicities of docetaxel are myelosuppression and edema. The edema is thought to be related to a capillary leak syndrome, and its onset usually occurs after cumulative doses of the drug. Premedication with steroids seems to delay the onset and ameliorate the severity of the edema associated with docetaxel. Both agents can also cause nausea and hair loss.

Bleomycin is an alkylating agent that causes single-strand DNA breaks. It is moderately effective as a single agent against squamous cell carcinoma of the head and neck and was extensively tested in combination with cisplatin and methotrexate. It is not commonly used today. Toxicities associated with bleomycin are pulmonary dysfunction (manifested initially as a decrease in carbon monoxide diffusion capacity), associated with cumulative doses over 400 U, and allergic reactions.

Methotrexate is still commonly used as a single agent for the palliation of recurrent or metastatic squamous cell carcinoma of the head and neck. Methotrexate is an antimetabolic agent and interferes with the activity of dihydrofolate reductase, an enzyme that catalyzes the carbon 1 (^1C) transfer reactions necessary for the synthesis of DNA bases. Methotrexate is usually administered on a weekly schedule as an intravenous bolus for palliative treatment of squamous cell carcinoma of the head and neck. The dose is usually between 40 and 60 mg/m^2, adjusted to the tolerance of the patient. The response rate is usually very low, less than 20%, and responses are usually short. Methotrexate has very little toxicity when administered on this schedule, although mild to moderate mucositis and/or myelosuppression can occur. Methotrexate should be used with caution in patients with renal dysfunction. It should not be used in patients with ascites or pleural effusion, because it tends to accumulate in these "third spaces," with a resultant increase in toxicities.

Organ preservation

Since the 1980s, there has been an effort to design treatments that would not require debilitating surgery, particularly laryngopharyngectomy, for patients with large tumors of the larynx and oropharynx. To date, these regimens have used two or more courses of cisplatin and continuous infusion of 5FU, followed by standard radiation therapy. Because these methods have resulted in preservation of the larynx in a significant number of patients without compromising the survival rate obtained with standard surgery and radiation, enthusiasm is high for developing new regimens that may even increase the cure rate, while preserving function.

In 1991, the Department of Veterans Affairs Laryngeal Cancer Study Group[5] reported its experience. This group randomized 332 patients with stage III and stage IV squamous cell carcinoma of the larynx to standard treatment with surgery followed by radiation, or to induction chemotherapy followed by radiation. Chemotherapy consisted of two courses of cisplatin and 5FU given every 3 to 4 weeks. After the second course, patients were evaluated for response. If there was at least a partial response, patients received a third course of chemotherapy. About a month after the third course, patients were treated with standard daily radiation therapy. If there was not at least a partial response after two courses of chemotherapy, patients were treated with surgical resection followed by radiation therapy. The survival rate for the two groups was similar, and the chemoradiation arm resulted in a laryngeal preservation rate of 66%.

In 1996, Lefebvre et al[6] reported a study done by the European Organization for Research and Treatment of Cancer. They randomized 202 patients with squamous cell cancers of the pyriform sinus and hypopharyngeal aspect of the aryepiglottic fold to either the standard surgical resection followed by radiation therapy, or to two courses of cisplatin and 5FU as in the trial by Wolf et al.[5] Patients who had a complete clinical response at the primary site after two or three courses of chemotherapy went on to receive radiation therapy. Patients who did not have a complete response were treated with surgery followed by radiation therapy. As in the previous study, survival rates were similar for the two groups. The median survival time in the surgery group was 25 months, and in the induction chemotherapy group it was 44 months. Laryngeal preservation was successful for 64% of the surviving patients at 3 years.

With these encouraging results, and pilot results obtained with patients who have unresectable disease, efforts are under way to improve the efficacy of organ preservation treatment as well as to diminish the short- and long-term toxicities associated with these treatments. A current intergroup trial in the United States randomizes patients with advanced laryngeal cancer to radiation therapy alone (not studied in the previous trials), versus radiation with concurrent cisplatin given every 3 weeks, versus induction chemotherapy with cisplatin and 5FU followed by radiation therapy. European trials in laryngeal and hypopharyngeal cancers will investigate induction chemotherapy followed by radiation versus different radiation schedules with or without concurrent chemotherapy.

Neoadjuvant and adjuvant chemotherapy

Cisplatin with 5FU can produce responses in up to 90% of patients who have not received prior therapy. Therefore, it seems attractive to try to shrink the tumor prior to definitive radiation or surgery. However, to date, this approach remains experimental, and reported studies have not shown an increase in survival rates with the use of neoadjuvant chemotherapy.[7,8]

Adjuvant chemotherapy after definitive surgery in patients with resectable squamous cell carcinoma of the head and neck may be useful in decreasing the probability of metastatic disease and may have an effect on local recurrence.[9,10] Patients with certain disease characteristics, such as extracapsular lymph node spread, multiple nodes, or positive margins, may benefit from this approach. Currently, adjuvant chemotherapy remains experimental, and a large national trial is randomizing such high-risk patients to either standard postoperative radiation therapy or postoperative radiation therapy with concurrent cisplatin treatment.

Local delivery of chemotherapy

Selective intra-arterial infusion of cisplatin, with or without concurrent radiation, has resulted in a response rate of approximately 90% in some tumors.[11,12] There is usually little systemic toxicity because of the local delivery of the drug and the simultaneous intravenous administration of an agent that counteracts cisplatin toxicity. However, this treatment has only been used in a select group of patients and requires an experienced medical and radiation oncologist, as well as an experienced interventional radiologist. Therefore, this approach remains experimental.

Chemotherapy for palliation

When cancers of the head and neck recur, and cannot be cured with surgery or radiation, when they are nonresponsive to initial management, or when the tumor metastasizes, the disease is incurable. However, palliative chemotherapy is sometimes helpful in improving quality of life by preventing or delaying pain and infection, which usually accompanies large locoregional recurrences. The oncologist must consider the factors previously noted, as well as the patient's goals, before deciding on a course of treatment. To date, combinations of agents have been shown to have higher response rates than single agents, but there is no significant impact on survival rates compared to a single agent.[13,14] The most common regimens used in palliative treatment are weekly methotrexate, cisplatin every 3 to 4 weeks, or a combination of cisplatin and 5FU. Paclitaxel has a 40% response rate as a single agent when given as a 24-hour infusion.[15] However, this regimen produces severe myelosuppression, requiring hematopoietic growth factors. Regimens including paclitaxel and cisplatin, paclitaxel and carboplatin, and docetaxel with cisplatin and/or 5FU are currently under evaluation in this population of patients.

Unresectable disease

Recently, therapy for locally advanced, unresectable disease has focused on combining chemotherapy with radiation therapy. While some centers still use induction chemotherapy followed by radiation, newer treatments have included concomitant chemotherapy and radiation. Recent studies have shown that concomitant administration may be more efficacious than the sequential approach.[8,16] Of course, concomitant administration of chemotherapy and radiation therapy is much more toxic than sequential administration. Patients must be observed closely, preferably by a multidisciplinary team, because most develop severe mucositis, and many experience dehydration and compromised nutrition. Weight loss of 6% to 10% is not unusual with these regimens. Most centers urge the patient to have a gastric tube placed prior to beginning treatment, which facilitates maintenance of adequate nutrition and hydration. The treatment takes 7 to 8 weeks, with a further 4 to 8 weeks of recovery, sometimes much longer. Some patients never fully recover swallowing function, and dry mouth from radiation damage to salivary glands can be a debilitating problem.

Patients with unresectable squamous cell carcinoma of the head and neck are sometimes debilitated and have sustained significant weight loss prior to diagnosis. In addition, they may have other comorbidities, most commonly chronic obstructive pulmonary disease, liver dysfunction, and coronary artery disease. Compromised swallowing function can lead to aspiration and pneumonias, sometimes with a fatal outcome, especially if pneumonia occurs when the white blood cell count is depressed after chemotherapy.

Despite the challenges of treating these patients, several promising studies have shown increased response rates in the 90% range, with 40% to 50% complete responses. Some regimens have involved induction chemotherapy followed by radiation with chemotherapy.[17] Other promising regimens have used weekly or longer infusions of paclitaxel with concurrent radiation, or have used weekly low-dose carboplatin plus paclitaxel in combination with radiation therapy.[3,18] Chemotherapy has also been used in rapidly alternating fashion with radiation therapy, and different administration schedules of radiation—with or without chemotherapy—have shown promising results.[19] Currently, concomitant chemoradiation therapy of some type is favored, but there is no single standard.

Nasopharyngeal cancer

Nasopharyngeal cancer usually presents at an advanced, inoperable stage. Several recent trials have demonstrated that chemotherapy and radiation can be curative for these cancers. Al-Sarraf et al[20] reported a trial that compared radiation therapy alone to concomitant cisplatin (every 3 weeks) and radiation therapy. Radiation therapy was to be followed by 3 courses of cisplatin and 5FU in the experimental group. The trial closed early because of significant disease-free survival rates and an overall survival benefit in the combined modality group. Similar findings have been reported from trials in Europe and Africa, with chemotherapy followed by radiation producing better disease-free survival rates, but not overall survival rates, compared to radiation therapy alone.[21]

Future Directions

Researchers will undoubtedly continue to discover more efficacious agents for the treatment of squamous cell carcinoma of the head and neck, as well as the best methods for combining modalities to effect longer and better survival. Although current regimens show promise, organ preservation approaches are accompanied by severe acute toxicity as well as debilitating late toxicity in a significant portion of patients. Agents that can decrease the toxicity of current treatments as well as enhance their activity are under evaluation. Newer agents, aimed at inhibition of metastasis, may also prove efficacious. Efforts to decrease the use of alcohol and tobacco must continue, and research into other factors that promote carcinoma in this region should be supported.

Summary

The use of chemotherapy to treat patients with squamous cell carcinoma of the head and neck has become common. Combined modality treatments, using chemotherapy and radiation, sometimes with surgery, are being studied to assess their efficacy in patients with unresectable disease, as well as for organ preservation. It is likely that such regimens, now currently being evaluated for laryngeal and oropharyngeal tumors, will also be evaluated for larger oral cancers. Research is ongoing for agents that will prolong and improve the response obtained with traditional chemotherapy agents.

References

1. Calvert AH, Newell DR, Gumbrell LA, O'Reilly S, Burnell M, Boxall FE, et al. Carboplatin dosage: Prospective evaluation of a simple formula based on renal function. J Clin Oncol 1989;11:1748–1756.

2. Rosenthal DI, Garth L, Lucci JA III, Schold SC, Truelson J, Fathallah-Skaykh H, et al. Phase I studies of continuous infusion paclitaxel given with standard aggressive radiation therapy for locally advanced solid tumors. Semin Oncol 1995;4:13–17.

3. Conley B, Jacobs M, Suntharalingam M, Zacharsky D, Ord RA, Gray W, et al. The role of paclitaxel/carboplatin and concurrent radiotherapy in unresectable squamous cell carcinoma of the head and neck: Recent findings. Semin Radiat Oncol 1997;7:S1–39.

4. Rowinsky EK, Donehower RC. Paclitaxel (Taxol). N Engl J Med 1995;332:1004.

5. The Department of Veterans Affairs Laryngeal Cancer Study Group. Induction chemotherapy plus radiation compared with surgery plus radiation in patients with advanced laryngeal cancer. N Engl J Med 1991;324:1685.

6. Lefebvre J-L, Chevalier D, Luboinski B, Kirkpatrick A, Collette L, Sahmoud T. Larynx preservation in pyriform sinus cancer: Preliminary results of a European Organization for Research and Treatment of Cancer phase III trial. J Natl Cancer Inst 1996;88:890.

7. Dimery IW, Hong WK. Combined modality therapies for head and neck cancer. J Natl Cancer Inst 1993;85:95.

8. El-Sayed S, Nelson N. Adjuvant and adjunctive chemotherapy in the management of squamous cell carcinoma of the head and neck region: A meta-analysis of prospective and randomized trials. J Clin Oncol 1996;14:838.

9. Cooper JS, Pajak TF, Forestiere A, Jacobs J, Fu KK, Ang KK, et al. Precisely defining high-risk operable head and neck tumors based on RTOG #85-03 and #88-24: Targets for postoperative radiochemotherapy. Head Neck 1998;20:588–594.

10. Laramore GE, Scott CV, Al-Sarraf M, Haselow RE, Ervin TJ, Wheeler R, et al. Adjuvant chemotherapy for resectable squamous cell carcinomas of the head and neck: Report on intergroup study 0034. Int J Radiat Oncol Biol Phys 1992;23:705–713.

11. Robbins KT, Storniolo AM, Kerber C, Vicario D, Seagren S, Shea M, et al. Phase I study of highly selective supradose cisplatin infusions for advanced head and neck cancer. J Clin Oncol 1994;12:2113–2120.

12. Robbins KT, Kumar P, Regine WF, Wong FS, Weir AB III, Flick P, et al. Efficacy of targeted supradose cisplatin and concomitant radiation therapy for advanced head and neck cancer: The Memphis experience. Int J Radiat Oncol Biol Phys 1997;8:263–271.

13. Jacobs C, Lyman G, Velez-Garcia E, Sridhar KS, Knight W, Hochster H, et al. A phase III randomized study comparing cisplatin and fluorouracil as single agents and in combination for advanced squamous cell carcinoma of the head and neck. J Clin Oncol 1992; 10:257–263.

14. Forastiere AA, Metch B, Schuller DE, Ensley JF, Hutchins LF, Triozzi P, et al. Randomized comparison of cisplatin plus fluorouracil and carboplatin plus fluorouracil versus methotrexate in advanced squamous cell carcinoma of the head and neck: A Southwest Oncology Group study. J Clin Oncol 1992;10: 1245–1251.

15. Forastiere AA, Neuberg D, Taylor SG, DeConti R, Adams G. Phase II evaluation of taxol in advanced head and neck cancer: An Eastern Cooperative Oncology Group trial. Monogr Natl Cancer Inst 1993;15:181.

16. Vokes EE, Weichselbaum RR. Concomitant chemoradiotherapy: Rationale and clinical experience in patients with solid tumors. J Clin Oncol 1990;8:911.

17. Vokes EE, Kies M, Haraf DJ, Mick R, Moran WJ, Kozloff M, et al. Induction chemotherapy followed by concomitant chemoradiotherapy for advanced head and neck cancer. Impact on the natural history of the disease. J Clin Oncol 1995;13:876–883.

18. Chougule P, Wanebo H, Akerley W, McRae R, Nigri P, Leone L, et al. Concurrent paclitaxel, carboplatin and radiotherapy in advanced head and neck cancers: A phase II study—preliminary results. Semin Oncol 1997;24:S19-57 to S19-61.

19. Leyvrax S, Pasche P, Bauer J, Bernasconi S, Monnier P. Rapidly alternating chemotherapy and hyperfractionated radiotherapy in the management of locally advanced head and neck carcinoma: Four-year results of a phase I/II study. J Clin Oncol 1994;12:1876.

20. Al-Sarraf M, LeBlanc M, Giri PG, Fu KK, Cooper J, Vuong T, et al. Chemoradiotherapy versus radiotherapy in patients with advanced nasopharyngeal cancer: Phase III randomized intergroup study 0099. J Clin Oncol 1998;16:1310–1317.

21. El Gueddari and International Nasopharynx Cancer Study Group. Final results of the VUMCA I randomized trial comparing neoadjuvant chemotherapy (BEC) plus radiotherapy (RT) to RT alone in undifferentiated nasopharyngeal carcinoma. Proc Am Soc Clin Oncol 1998;17:385a.

PART III

Rehabilitation

CHAPTER 11

Oral Care of the Patient Receiving Chemotherapy

Miriam R. Robbins, DDS, MS

The oral cavity is a frequent site of the side effects of aggressive chemotherapy, with acute and chronic oral complications developing in 40% to 75% of patients receiving treatment.[1-3] Significant risk factors for the development of oral complications include the type of malignancy, the chemotherapeutic agents used, the cumulative dose, the method of delivery, and the degree and duration of myelosuppression. Poorly maintained dentition, oral and dental disease, moderate to advanced periodontal disease, ill-fitting prostheses, and inadequate oral care during treatment increase the severity of complications.[4-7]

All chemotherapeutic agents damage rapidly dividing cells. The mucosal membranes of the oral cavity have rapid epithelial turnover, rendering them vulnerable to the effects of cytotoxic agents.[8] Direct cytotoxicity results in interruption of the integrity of the mucosa and in an increased risk for local or systemic infection in the immunosuppressed patient.[9-12]

Oral complications resulting from anticancer therapies significantly affect morbidity, the patient's ability to tolerate treatment, and the overall quality of life.[13] The objective of care for the patient is to prevent or decrease oral complications and to modify the acute and long-term consequences of the therapy.[7]

Oral Complications

Mucositis/stomatitis

Direct stomatotoxicity or mucositis, a result of the cytotoxic effect on the cells, is the most common acute oral complication of chemotherapy.[14] It may be seen as early as 3 days or, more commonly, 5 to 7 days after the start of treatment. To date, chemotherapy-induced mucositis is most frequently seen with cyclophosphamide, bleomycin, cytarabine (ara-C), doxorubicin, daunorubicin (Adriamycin), etoposide, 5-fluorouracil, methotrexate, mitomycin, mercaptopurine, vinblastine, vincristine, and floxuridine.[15] Conditioning regimens for bone marrow transplants, continuous infusion, or frequent repetitive schedules are more likely to cause mucositis than equivalent doses of similar drugs given in a single bolus.[9]

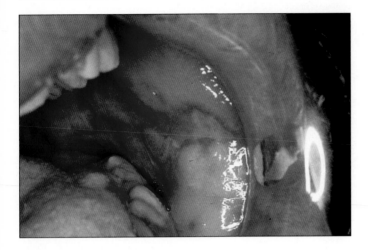

Fig 11-1 Oral ulcerations secondary to chemotherapy.

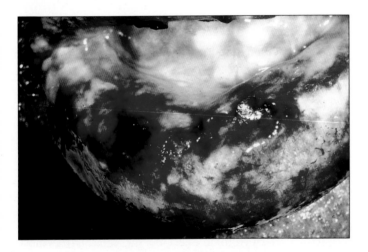

Fig 11-2 Severe mucositis secondary to a conditioning regimen for bone marrow transplant.

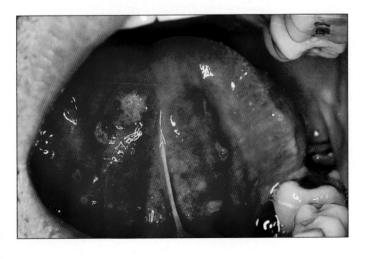

Fig 11-3 Oral ulcerations located on the ventral surface of the tongue and floor of the mouth following administration of vincristine.

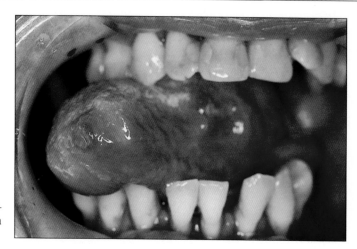

Fig 11-4 Ulceration of the lateral border of the tongue secondary to edema and mechanical trauma.

Chemotherapy causes a decrease in the renewal rate of the basal epithelium. This results in atrophy and thinning of the mucosa as well as the development of edema and erythematous burnlike lesions (Figs 11-1 to 11-3). These areas quickly ulcerate and coalesce to form large areas of mucosal denudation[16] covered with a whitish-gray membrane. Areas of deeper ulceration with erythematous halos and necrotic centers may develop, especially on the lips, ventral surface of the tongue, floor of the mouth, buccal mucosa, and soft palate.[17] Patients experience difficulty swallowing and eating due to severe pain, often resulting in decreased nutritional intake and dehydration.[18] Patients who develop mucositis during their initial cycle of chemotherapy usually continue to develop increasingly severe mucositis during subsequent cycles. Mucositis can become cumulative and is often the factor that limits the amount of chemotherapy that can be given, compromising treatment outcomes.[19]

Indirect stomatotoxicity, or stomatitis, refers to injury of the mucosal tissues by trauma (ie, biting, irritation from dental prosthe-

ses or orthodontic appliances) or infections. Although the terms *mucositis* and *stomatitis* are used interchangeably, stomatitis has a specific cause and treatment aimed at identifying and eliminating the precipitating factor,[20] whereas mucositis results from the direct effect of chemotherapy on cells. Factors that can initiate stomatitis include the presence of microorganisms, local mucosal health, and the balance between the patient's overall physical health and the suppressive action of the therapy. Edema of the buccal mucosa and tongue can lead to serration by the teeth[21] (Fig 11-4). Dentures can produce traumatic wounds while harboring microorganisms that can cause secondary infections. Reactivation of the herpes simplex virus (HSV) can also cause mucosal ulceration early in the chemotherapy cycle.[22]

Infectious stomatitis can occur indirectly from the myelosuppression caused by chemotherapy. It usually occurs 7 to 12 days after administration of an agent, corresponding to the nadir of the white blood cell count in the patient with neutropenia. Periodontal pockets and/or periapical pathosis may pro-

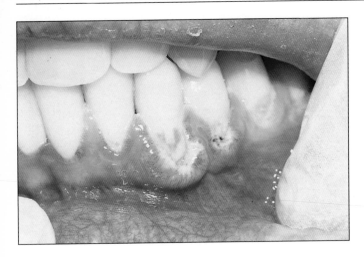

Fig 11-5 Breakdown of the marginal gingiva.

vide a reservoir of pathogenic and opportunistic organisms that cause local or systemic infections during periods of myelosuppression.[23,24] Marginal and papillary gingival inflammation can lead to breakdown of the gingiva, followed by ulcerative lesions that can extend to any region of the mucosa (Fig 11-5).

Infections

Oral infections in the immunosuppressed patient can become life-threatening. The incidence of infection varies with the type of malignancy, degree of myelosuppression, and host susceptibility.[25] In hematologic malignancies, 50% of oral infections are caused by *Candida albicans*, 25% by HSV, 15% by gram-negative bacilli, and 10% by gram-positive cocci.[26] Seventy percent of patients being treated for solid tumors have oral infections caused by fungi, 10% by HSV, 10% by gram-negative bacilli, and 10% by gram-positive cocci.[27] Although normal flora often is the cause of the infection, there is a shift in the oral flora in immunosuppressed patients toward gram-negative organisms (*Pseudomonas, Proteus, Escherichia coli,* and *Klebsiella*).[27] Underlying oral diseases, such as periodontitis, present an increase in anaerobes and spirochetes. Prolonged antimicrobial or corticosteroid therapy may encourage an overgrowth of opportunistic organisms.[28]

Fungi account for most of the oral infections, with *Candida albicans* causing both superficial and disseminated infections.[29] Sites most commonly affected include the tongue, buccal mucosa, palate, and pharyngeal mucosa (Fig 11-6). Candidal infections may present not only as pseudomembranous (removable white plaques) but also as hyperplastic (leukoplakia-like plaques that do not rub off), erythematous (patchy erythema), and angular cheilitis. The fungal colonies tend to coalesce and spread, covering extensive areas of the mucosal surface.[30]

Herpes simplex virus and herpes zoster (HSZ) are the most common viral pathogens causing infections in the patient receiving chemotherapy.[31] Reactivation of latent virus

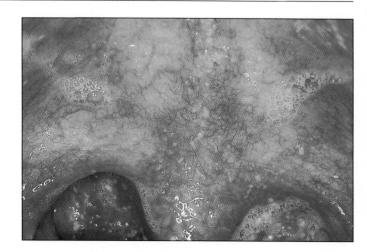

Fig 11-6 Candidiasis, a frequent cause of mucosal infection in myelosuppressed patients.

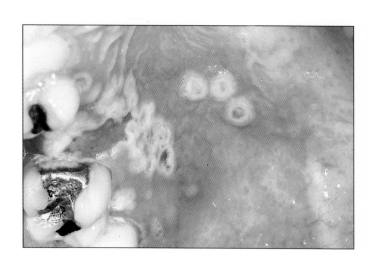

Fig 11-7 Ulceration of the palate caused by herpes simplex. Lesions may have an atypical appearance in immunosuppressed patients.

can cause herpetic gingivostomatitis and labialis. Lesions can occur on any oral or perioral surface (Fig 11-7). Symptoms of itching, burning, and pain are followed by vesicles that quickly rupture, leaving multiple ulcerations on an erythematous base. These lesions can mimic the ulcerations that develop as a result of the direct stomatotoxic effects of chemotherapy.[32] Lesions can enlarge peripherally, causing extensive necrosis. They can take a protracted time to resolve, especially in the patient with profound neutropenia.[25,33] Opportunistic superinfection may occur con-comitantly and is often a more serious threat than the viral infection alone.

Hemorrhage

Intraoral hemorrhage can be caused by treatment-induced thrombocytopenia and/or coagulopathy or by myelosuppression secondary to the neoplastic process.[23] Bleeding is uncommon when the platelet count is more than 50,000/mm^3, but the chance of spontaneous bleeding when the platelet count falls below

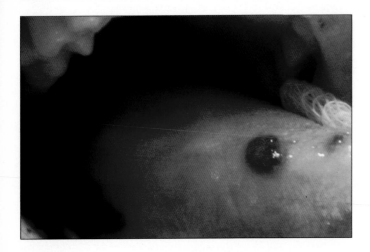

Fig 11-8 Small blood-filled blisters on the lateral border of the tongue of a patient receiving chemotherapy for breast cancer.

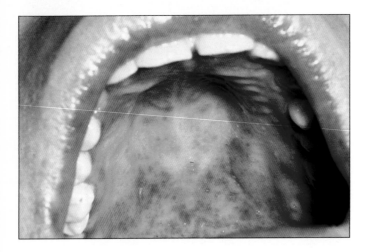

Fig 11-9 Petechiae located on the soft palate.

$20,000/mm^3$ exceeds 50%.[34] Petechiae on the palate and gingiva are the most common signs of decreased platelet counts (Figs 11-8 and 11-9). Underlying oral inflammation can exacerbate bleeding tendencies. Bleeding can occur spontaneously or be precipitated by minimal trauma from oral hygiene techniques, mobility secondary to periodontal disease, fractured restorations or teeth, dental prostheses, or orthodontic appliances. Bleeding is usually oozing and intermittent and can occur at multiple sites, making control difficult.[27] Clots are often friable and easily disrupted.

Treatment usually includes transfusion of platelets or coagulation factors until the bone marrow recovers.

Xerostomia

Quality and quantity of saliva can be reduced as early as 2 days after the administration of some chemotherapeutic agents (particularly doxorubicin) or as a result of other medications the patient may be taking. The duration of therapy can contribute to the degree of xerostomia. Patients may complain of general dryness and develop thick, ropy saliva, probably as a result of cytotoxic effects on the parotid glands. There is a decreased salivary pH and a shift in the oral flora toward more cariogenic species.[35] Loss of protective immunoproteins coupled with the increased acidity and the presence of cariogenic microorganisms can often lead to an accelerated rate of decay similar to radiation caries.[36] An increased rate of candidal overgrowth is also related to decreased salivary flow. Xerostomia can make mucosal surfaces more susceptible to trauma and subsequent ulceration and exacerbate existing mucositis. With the exception of the bone marrow transplant patients who develop chronic graft-versus-host disease, chemotherapy-induced xerostomia is transient and resolves upon cessation of chemotherapy.[21]

Neurotoxicity

Some chemotherapeutic agents (particularly the plant alkaloids vincristine and vinblastine) can cause neurotoxicity, with nerve damage closely related to total dose and duration of therapy.[37] The neurotoxic effects usually manifest as pain and/or neuropathy of the extremities. Involvement of the cranial nerves can produce altered sensation, causalgia, or partial paresthesia of the perioral and intraoral areas innervated by the trigeminal nerve.[38] Patients can experience severe, bilateral throbbing pain that mimics that of odontogenic or periodontal origin, especially in the region of the mandibular molars. The diagnosis of neurotoxicity is difficult and complicated by the fact that the symptoms may resolve spontaneously, only to return with increased intensity. The absence of clinical or radiographic odontogenic or periodontal pathosis, knowledge of the patient's drug regimen, and the presence of bilateral pain can aid in identifying the cause.

Treatment involves the use of systemic analgesics, usually narcotics. Pain resolves when the chemotherapy is discontinued, although residual neuropathy may remain.

Dental Treatment Prior to Chemotherapy

Pretreatment evaluation

A prechemotherapy dental evaluation, preventive care, and intense oral hygiene instruction should be part of a patient's initial workup. The initial examination should include a thorough head and neck examination, oral and dental examinations, and radiographic evaluation aimed at documenting acute and chronic conditions that could produce or exacerbate complications. Potential sources of infection (ie, plaque, calculus, periapical pathosis, acute dental abscesses, periodontal disease, caries, partially impacted third molars) and irritations (ie, defective restorations, ill-fitting prostheses) should be carefully evaluated. Resolving these problems prior to initiation of therapy helps to decrease oral complications and prevent the development of local or systemic infection.[5,39,40]

Teeth with acute abscesses or symptomatic periapical pathologic conditions, nonrestorable teeth, and teeth with severe periodontal involvement should be extracted at least 10 days prior to an anticipated neutrophil count of less than 1,000/mm³ after consultation with the oncologist.[41] Alveolectomy and primary wound closure should be obtained. Because hemostatic packing agents (eg, Gelfoam, Surgicel) provide a good culture medium for bacterial and fungal growth, they are contraindicated.[42] Prophylactic antibiotics should be given if the absolute neutrophil count is less than 2,000/mm³. If there is

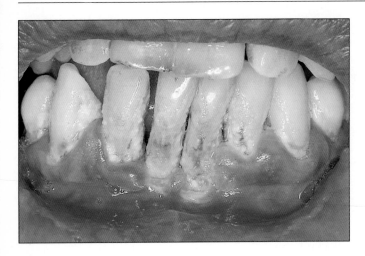

Fig 11-10 Acute periodontal infection with necrotic hard and soft tissue following treatment for leukemia.

not enough time to extract teeth with significant periapical pathosis or symptomatic pulpal involvement, pulpal therapy should be initiated prior to chemotherapy to eliminate a reservoir of virulent microbes. However, endodontic therapy should only be performed if there is at least a 7-day interval between the treatment and profound myelosuppression (neutrophil counts < 1,000/mm³). Extraction can then be performed as soon as the hematologic status allows.[42]

Caries should be removed to decrease the presence of bacteria intraorally. Rough or sharp tooth surfaces should be smoothed to decrease soft tissue trauma. Orthodontic brackets must be removed. In children, all mobile primary teeth should be removed as well as those that are expected to be exfoliated during treatment to prevent bleeding.

For patients expected to have profound or prolonged nadir counts, soft vinyl mouthguards can be used in controlling hemorrhage or infection. Topical hemostatic, antifungal, antiviral, and anesthetic agents can be placed in the mouthguard to ensure increased contact between oral tissues and the medications.[43]

Oral hygiene

Plaque can become a source of bacteremia. As gingivitis is allowed to progress, inflammation can lead to bleeding and ulceration, providing a portal for local and systemic infection (Fig 11-10).[44] A major objective prior to and during chemotherapy is to educate the patient about the importance of maintaining excellent oral hygiene, keeping the development of plaque and calculus to an absolute minimum. The dental team must see the patient on a frequent recall schedule to maintain a clean oral cavity and to reinforce patient education. Patients need to be aware of the benefits of controlling plaque and thereby bacteremia and that these benefits outweigh the risk posed by the transient bacteremia produced by brushing. If the patient's platelet counts drop below 40,000/mm³, flossing should be discontinued, but oral hygiene needs to be continued using an ultrasoft "chemobrush" to reduce bleeding from toothbrush trauma.[44] Foam brushes (Toothettes), oral irrigation, or swishing fluids are not adequate to remove plaque and debris.[5]

Gentle rinses using a solution of salt (2.5 mL), sodium bicarbonate (10 mL), and warm water (0.95 L) aid in the removal of superficial food debris, dilute bacterial counts, soothe irritated tissues, and decrease acidity in the oral cavity. These should be done at least four times a day and followed with a water rinse. Commercial mouthrinses containing alcohol and/or phenol can further desiccate the oral mucosa. This increases mucosal susceptibility to ulceration and is poorly tolerated if ulcerated areas are already present. Very dilute solutions of hydrogen peroxide (30 mL 3% peroxide to 240 mL water) followed by a water rinse can be effective in cleansing the tissues of mucus and crusted material.[45] Peroxide should not be used in patients with mucositis, because it inhibits reepithialization. It also cannot be used when there are blood clots or bleeding, because it precipitates more bleeding. Chlorhexidine, effective against gram-positive bacilli, yeast, and other fungi, can be used to reduce the microbial population in the oral cavity.[7] However, most commercial preparations have an alcohol content of at least 9.6%, which makes them poorly tolerated in patients with mucositis. Chlorhexidine diluted with warm water retains some antimicrobial activity and is more comfortable to use. However, it should not be used concurrently with nystatin, which decreases the antimicrobial effectiveness.

To help maintain cleanliness, edentulous patients should clean their mouths with moist gauze and use frequent rinses, especially after meals. Toothettes soaked in chlorhexadine can be used to clean the alveolar ridges, palate, and tongue.[46,47] Dentures should be left out as much as possible to decrease mucosal irritation. All dental prostheses must be thoroughly cleaned daily and soaked in either a commercial denture cleaner or a nystatin solution to prevent infections.

Dental Treatment During Chemotherapy

Patients are at an increased risk of infection after chemotherapy is initiated. Any dental treatment should only be done after consultation with the patient's oncologist to coordinate treatment with the patient's optimal hematologic status. A white blood cell count greater than 1,000/mm^3 and a platelet count greater than 40,000/mm^3 with a normal coagulation profile are necessary prior to any dental treatment.[48] Antibiotic prophylaxis is required when the absolute neutrophil count is less than 2,000/mm^3.[42] Patients with indwelling catheters also require prophylactic antibiotic coverage. The optimal time to perform dental treatment is just prior to a cycle of chemotherapy, maximizing the time before nadir is expected. At any time, symptomatic teeth with pulpal involvement can be opened, debrided, and closed with a temporary restoration. Decay can be excavated and sedative fillings placed. Generally, extractions are contraindicated, except in extreme emergencies when an infected tooth can be the source of systemic infection.

Treatment of Complications

Mucositis

Since there are currently no good preventive approaches available, management of mucositis is primarily palliative. Patients should be advised to eat a soft, bland diet and to avoid hard, abrasive foods that can mechanically traumatize the tissues. The oral mucosa should be cleaned as atraumatically as possible with an ultrasoft toothbrush or wet gauze. Sodium bicarbonate rinses used frequently clean and lubricate tissues, prevent crusting, and soothe sore tissues. In mild cases, dilute chlorhexidine rinses can be used to decrease oral microflora. For increased penetration of topical medication, tissues must be cleaned of mucus and debris prior to application. Following emesis, patients should rinse their mouth with sodium bicarbonate solution and swallow some water to clear the throat of acidic secretions. These secretions can cause increased irritation and ulceration of the mucosa.

Suspensions of topical anesthetics can be used to alleviate discomfort. Topical anesthetics, such as dyclonine hydrochloride (0.5%) and viscous lidocaine hydrochloride (2%) solution, can be effective in relieving discomfort but also can be chemically irritating. Care must be taken not to mechanically traumatize anesthetized tissues.[49] A 1:2 dilution with water decreases the profound numbing effect and can still provide relief. Topical anesthetics can be combined with coating agents like magnesium hydroxide (milk of magnesia, Maalox) or kaolin-pectin (Kaopectate) and diphenhydramine hydrochloride (Benadryl elixir) elixir in a 1:4:4 mixture to produce a swish-and-expectorate or swallow rinse.[50] A cool solution can increase relief; thus, refrigerating or freezing the solution into ice cubes to dissolve in the mouth is recommended.

Sucralfate, an antiulcer drug, binds to ulcerated tissue by attaching to proteins in the damaged mucosa. It forms an adhesive-like protective coating. Available in tablet form, it can be dissolved in water to make a rinse.[51] Dyclonine or lidocaine can be added to the solution to decrease pain and can be swished and expectorated or swallowed up to six times per day.[52]

Zilactin is a medicated gel that contains tannic acid and forms an occlusive film over oral ulcerations. It must be applied to dried tissue, which often causes increased discomfort and decreases patient acceptance.[53]

Kamillosan Liquidim (from the flower of the chamomile plant) rinse (10 to 15 drops dissolved in 120 mL of warm water) can be used three times a day. Its main ingredients (chamazulene, levomenol, polyins, and flavonoids) are thought to have anti-inflammatory, spasmolytic, and antibacterial action and help promote granulation and reepithelization of ulcerated tissues.[54]

Cryotherapy, in the form of ice chips, used for 5 minutes prior to drug administration and for 25 minutes afterward, can decrease the mucositis associated with 5-fluorouracil, possibly by causing local vasoconstriction and reducing local delivery of the agent.[55] Allopurinol rinses have been shown to be effective in protecting against methotrexate-induced mucositis.[56]

In the future, the control of mucositis may be found in cellular engineering and manipulation. Cytokine-stimulated neutrophil recovery using agents such as granulocyte colony-stimulating factor and granulocyte-macrophage colony-stimulating factors decreases the duration of mucositis either by limiting epithelial damage or by decreasing the likelihood of secondary infection and delayed healing.[57,58] Transforming growth factor–beta 3 and interleukin-2 have demonstrated promising efficacy by transiently limiting the rate of basal oral epithelial growth proliferation in vitro and in vivo, thereby modifying the frequency and severity of chemotherapy-induced mucositis.[59,60]

Infections

Many patients are treated prophylactically against fungal infection if their neutrophil counts are less than 1,500/mm^3.[6] Topical or systemic agents can be used depending on the

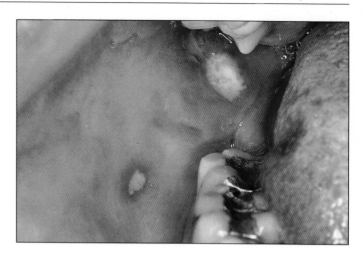

Fig 11-11 Ulcerations secondarily infected with gram-negative bacteria.

degree of immunosuppression. Topical nystatin rinses (100,000 U 4 times a day) or chlortrimazole troches (10 mg 5 times a day) are typically effective.[61] With decreased salivary flow, troches may not readily dissolve and solutions may be preferable. Patients should be instructed to thoroughly clean the oral cavity prior to taking any antifungal medications. Dental prostheses should be removed, to allow medication to reach all intraoral tissues, and treated to prevent reinfection. Toothbrushes should be disinfected after each use.

Bacterial infections can be a major cause of morbidity and mortality in immunocompromised patients. Erythema and other inflammatory signs may be suppressed intraorally, especially in patients with bone marrow transplants (Fig 11-11). When there are systemic signs of infection or areas of chronic disease or pain, specimens of these areas should be cultured to determine the presence of pathogenic organisms.[62] Broad-spectrum antibiotics are usually indicated at the first

sign of infection to reduce the danger of gram-negative sepsis.[63] Patients with neutrophil counts of less than 1,000/mm³ need intravenous broad-spectrum antibiotics. Depending on the patient's hematologic status, definitive surgical interventions such as incision and drainage, extraction, or periodontal debridement can be initiated once the patient has been stabilized. Platelet transfusions may be necessary if platelet counts are less than 50,000/mm³.

Viral infections are generally treated with acyclovir, either orally or intravenously. If a patient is known to be at risk for HSV reactivation due to seropositivity and prolonged myelosuppression, treatment is generally started prophylactically. Early recognition of HSV infection is important so that treatment can be initiated. Because HSV lesions are frequently mistaken for chemotherapy-induced mucositis, culturing can aid in differentiating between the two. Herpetic lesions that become secondarily infected with fungus or bacteria require combined treatments (Fig 11-12).

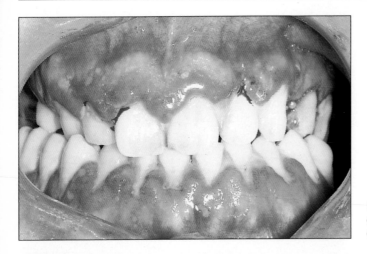

Fig 11-12 Patient with herpetic gingivostomatitis secondarily infected by oral bacteria.

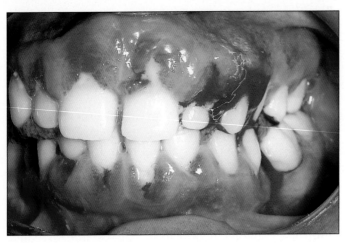

Fig 11-13 Gingival bleeding in a patient with acute leukemia and decreased platelet count.

Hemorrhage

Prevention is the best approach to avoid hemorrhage. Maintaining good oral hygiene and eliminating marginal gingivitis can help decrease the chance of bleeding in a patient with thrombocytopenia (Fig 11-13). Daily rinsing with chlorhexidine is effective in reducing inflammation.[64] When bleeding occurs, application of periodontal dressing and local coagulants such as topical thrombin can be used. Transfusions of platelets, whole blood, or plasma may be necessary. In patients with profound bone marrow suppression (patients with hematologic malignancies or those undergoing bone marrow transplant), soft vinyl mouthguards can be lined with Xerofoam sprinkled with Avitene, or filled with Gelfoam or Surgicel sprinkled with topical thrombin, and placed over the teeth and soft tissue. These can be removed every 8 hours, cleaned, and replaced with a fresh liner. Vigorous mouthrinses should be discouraged to avoid dislodgment of clots. The patient should eat a soft diet to avoid mechanical chemical trauma, which may reinitiate bleeding.[23]

Xerostomia

Frequent rinses help to hydrate the mucosa. Patients should be encouraged to drink plenty of liquids, to avoid smoking and alcohol, and to use sugarless gum or candy as a salivary stimulant. Dried lips can be coated with a lubricant containing lanolin or cocoa butter. Petroleum jelly should be avoided as it can promote bacterial growth. Moisturizing gels and artificial saliva preparations containing carboxymethylcellulose or hydroxyethylcellulose, such as OralBalance, Xerolube, or Oralube, can be used. For dentate patients with prolonged xerostomia, neutral pH 1.1% sodium fluoride gel can be used daily to prevent the development of chemocaries until the completion of treatment.

Dental Treatment Following Chemotherapy

Chances of complications from dental treatments are decreased during remission. Therefore, regular dental examinations and routine oral hygiene sessions are imperative. Restorative, endodontic, periodontal, and exodontic procedures should be performed promptly to alleviate any potential dental problems during subsequent episodes of illness and therapy.

Summary

The primary goal of dental management is to prevent complications caused by chemotherapy and its resultant immunosuppression. An emphasis on prophylactic measures prior to therapy can decrease the morbidity of therapy and greatly enhance the patient's quality of life. Early dental intervention and elimination of problems prior to chemotherapy can minimize oral complications.

References

1. DeVita VT. Principles of cancer management. In: DeVita VT, Hellman S, Roseberg SA (eds). Cancer: Principles and Practice of Oncology, ed 5. Philadelphia: Lippincott-Raven, 1997:307–332.

2. Sonis ST. Oral complications of cancer therapy. In: DeVita VT, Hellman S, Rosenberg SA (eds). Cancer: Principles and Practice of Oncology, ed 5. Philadelphia: Lippincott-Raven, 1997:2385–2393.

3. Berger AM, Kilroy TJ. Oral complications. In: DeVita VT, Hellman S, Roseberg SA (eds). Cancer: Principles and Practice of Oncology, ed 5. Philadelphia: Lippincott-Raven, 1997:2714–2725.

4. Peterson DE. Oral toxicity of chemotherapeutic agents. Semin Oncol 1992;19:478–491.

5. Toth BB, Chambers MS, Fleming JC, Martin JW. Minimizing oral complications of cancer treatment. Oncology 1995;9:851–866.

6. Carl W. Oral complications of local and systemic cancer treatment. Curr Opin Oncol 1995;7:320–324.

7. Toth BB, Chambers MS, Fleming TC. Prevention and management of oral complications associated with cancer therapies: Radiotherapy/chemotherapy. Tex Dent J 1996;113:23–29.

8. Toth BB, Martin JW, Fleming TC. Oral complications associated with cancer therapy: M.D. Anderson Cancer Center experience. J Clin Periodontol 1990;17:508–515.

9. Sonis ST, Clark J. Prevention and management of oral mucositis induced by antineoplastic therapy. Oncology 1991;5:11–18.

10. Dreizen S, Bodey GP, Rodriquez V. Oral complications of cancer chemotherapy. Postgrad Med 1975;58:75–79.

11. Singh N, Scully C, Joyston-Bechal S. Oral complications of cancer therapies: Preventions and management. Clin Oncol 1996;8:15–24.

12. Dodd M, Facione N, Dibble S, MacPhail L. Comparison of methods to determine the prevalence and nature of oral mucositis. Cancer Pract 1996;4:312–318.

13. Consensus statement: Oral complications of cancer therapy. NCI Monogr 1990;9:3–8.

14. Peterson D, D'Ambrosio J. Diagnosis and management of acute and chronic oral complications of nonsurgical cancer therapies. Dent Clin North Am 1992;36: 945–966.

15. Guggenheimer J, Vebin RS, Appel BN, et al. Clinicopathologic effects of cancer chemotherapy agents on human mucosa. Oral Surg Oral Med Oral Pathol 1977;44:58–63.

16. Toth BB, Martin JW, Fleming TJ. Oral and dental care associated with cancer therapy. Cancer Bull 1991;43:397–402.

17. Barrett AP. Gingival lesions in leukemia: A classification. J Periodontol 1984;55:586–588.

18. Minasian A, Dwyer J. Nutritional implications of dental and swallowing issues in head and neck cancer. Oncology 1998;12:1155–1169.

19. Miaskowski C. Management of mucositis during therapy. NCI Monogr 1990;9:95–97.

20. Ziga S. Stomatitis/mucositis. In: Yasko J (ed). Guidelines for Cancer Care: Symptom Management. Reston, VA: Reston, 1983:213–223.

21. Carl W, Sako K. Cancer and the Oral Cavity. Chicago: Quintessence, 1986:151–167.

22. Scully C, Epstein J. Oral health care for the cancer patient. Eur J Cancer B Oral Oncol 1996;32B: 281–292.

23. Rosenberg SW. Oral care of the chemotherapy patient. Dent Clin North Am 1990;34:239–250.

24. Meurman JH, Pryhonrn S, Teerenhovi L, Lindquist C. Oral sources of septicaemia in patients with malignancies. Oral Oncol 1997;33:389–397.

25. Dreizen S. Description and incidence of oral complications. NCI Monogr 1990;9:11–15.

26. Martin MV, van Saene HK. The role of oral microorganisms in cancer therapy. Curr Opin Dent 1992;2: 81–84.

27. Mealy BL, Semba SE, Hallman WW. Dentistry and the cancer patient: Part I. Oral manifestations and complications of chemotherapy. Compend Contin Educ Dent 1994;15:1252–1261.

28. Wingard JR. Infectious and noninfectious systemic consequences. NCI Monogr 1990;9:21–26.

29. Ostchega Y. Preventing and treating cancer chemotherapy's oral complications. Nursing 1980;10:47–52.

30. Dreizen S, Bodey GP, Valdivieso M. Chemotherapy-associated oral infections in adults with solid tumors. Oral Surg Oral Med Oral Pathol 1983;55:113–120.

31. Eisen D, Essel J, Broun E. Oral cavity complications of bone marrow transplantation. Semin Cutan Med Surg 1997;16:265–272.

32. Redding SW. Role of herpes simplex virus reactivation in chemotherapy-induced oral mucositis. NCI Monogr 1990;9:103–106.

33. Dreizen S, McCredie KB, Bodey GP, et al. Mucocutaneous herpetic infections during chemotherapy. Postgrad Med 1988;84:181–190.

34. Fattore L, Baer R, Olsen R. The role of the general dentist in the treatment and management of oral complications of chemotherapy. Gen Dent 1987;35:374–377.

35. Carl W. Managing the oral manifestation of cancer therapy. Part II. Chemotherapy. Compend Contin Educ Dent 1988;9:376–386.

36. Main BE, Calman KC, Ferguson MM, et al. The effects of cytotoxic therapy on saliva and oral flora. Oral Surg Oral Med Oral Pathol 1984;58:545–548.

37. Vuolo SJ. Oral complications of cancer chemotherapy and dental care for the cancer patient receiving antineoplastic drug therapy. N Y J Dent 1987;57:50–59.

38. McCarthy GM, Skillings JR. Jaw and other oralfacial pain in patients receiving vincristine for the treatment of cancer. Oral Surg Oral Med Oral Pathol 1992;74:229–304.

39. Sonis, ST. Pretreatment oral assessment. NCI Monogr 1990;9:29–32.

40. Sonis ST, Kunz A. Impact of improved dental services on the frequency of oral complications of cancer therapy. J Oral Surg 1988;65:19–22.

41. Overholser CD, Peterson DE, Bergman SA. Dental extractions in patients with acute nonlymphocytic leukemia. Oral Maxillofac Surg 1982;40:296–298.

42. Peterson DE. Pretreatment strategies for infection prevention in chemotherapy patients. NCI Monogr 1990;9:61–71.

43. McClure D, Baker G, Baker B, et al. Oral management of the cancer patient. Part I. Oral complications of chemotherapy. Compend Contin Educ Dent 1987;8: 41–50.

44. Peterson DE, Minah GE, Overholser CD, et al. Microbiology of acute periodontal infections in myelosuppressed cancer patients. J Clin Oncol 1987;5:1461–1468.

45. Addems A, Epstein JB, Damji S, et al. The lack of efficacy of a foam brush in maintaining gingival health: A controlled study. Spec Care Dentist 1992;12:103–106.

46. Ferretti G, Brown AT, Raybould TP, Lillich TT. Oral antimicrobial agents: Chlorhexadine. NCI Monogr 1990;9:51–55.

47. Epstein J, Ransier A, Lunn R, Spinelli J. Enhancing the effect of oral hygiene with the use of foam brushes with chlorhexadine. Oral Surg Oral Med Oral Pathol 1994;77:242–247.

48. Semba SE, Mealey BL, Hallmon WW. Dentistry and the cancer patient. Part 2. Oral health management of the chemotherapy patient. Compend Contin Educ Dent 1994;15:1378–1388.

49. McWherter JA, Herrin HK. Oral complications in the cancer patient. Tex Dent J 1996;113:39–42.

50. Barker G, Loftus L, Cuddy P, Barker B. The effects of sucralfate suspension and diphenhydramine syrup plus kaolin-pectin on radiation-induced mucositis. Oral Surg Oral Med Oral Pathol 1991;71:288–293.

51. Adams, Toth B, Dudly BS. Evaluation of sulcrafate suspension for the treatment of stomatitis. Clin Pharmacol Ther 1985;37:178–183.

52. Shenep JL, Kalwihsky DK, Hutson PR. Efficacy of oral sucralfate suspension in prevention and treatment of chemotherapy-induced mucositis. J Pediatr 1988;113:758–763.

53. Madeya ML. Oral complications from cancer therapy. Part 2. Nursing implications for assessment and treatment. Oncol Nurs Forum 1996;23:808–819.

54. Carl W, Emrich LS. Management of oral mucositis during local radiation and systemic chemotherapy: A study of 98 patients. J Prosthet Dent 1991;66:361–368.

55. Symonds RP. Treatment-induced mucositis: An old problem with new remedies. Br J Cancer 1998;77:1689–1695.

56. Mahood DJ, Dose AM, Loprinzi C. Inhibition of fluorouracil-induced stomatitis by oral cryotherapy. J Clin Oncol 1991;9:449–452.

57. Rosso M, Blasi G, Gherlone E, Rosso R. Effect of granulocyte-macrophage colony-stimulating factor on prevention of mucositis in head and neck patients treated with chemo-radiotherapy. J Chemother 1997;9:382–385.

58. Gabrilove JL, Jakubowski A, Scher H, et al. Effect of granulocyte colony stimulating factor on neutropenia and associated morbidity due to chemotherapy for transitional cell carcinoma of the urothelium. N Engl J Med 1988;318:1414–1422.

59. Sonis ST, Lindquist L, VanVugit A. Prevention of chemotherapy induced ulcerative mucositis by transforming growth factor beta-3. Cancer Res 1994;54:1135.

60. Keith JC, Albert L, Sonis ST, et al. IL-11: A pleiotropic cytokine: Exciting new effects of IL-11 on gastrointestinal mucosal biology. Stem Cells 1994;12:79.

61. Toth BB, Frame RT. Dental oncology: The management of disease and treatment related oral/dental complications associated with chemotherapy. Curr Probl Cancer 1983;7:7–35.

62. Shenep JL. Combination and single-agent empirical antibacterial therapy for febrile cancer patients with neutropenia and mucositis. NCI Monogr 1990;9:117–121.

63. Schimpff SC. Surveillance cultures. NCI Monogr 1990;9:37–42.

64. Nguyen AMH. Dental management of patients who receive chemo- and radiation therapy. Gen Dent 1992;40:305–311.

CHAPTER 12

Oral Care of the Patient Receiving Radiation Therapy

Miriam R. Robbins, DDS, MS

The reaction of the tissues of the head and neck, both perioral and oral, varies with the type of radiation used, area of exposure, dose given per fraction, time between fractions, duration of treatment, and total dose received. Radiation causes both acute and chronic tissue changes that have a profound effect on oral health during and after radiation therapy. Unlike chemotherapy, the transient effects of radiation therapy are chronic, irreversible, and progressive due to permanent damage to the proliferative cells of the head and neck.[1]

Acute oral sequelae include mucositis, taste alterations, infectious stomatitis, dermatitis, and dysphagia. The chronic, permanent changes include xerostomia, radiation caries, trismus, periodontal deterioration, decreased resiliency in perioral tissue, intrinsic bone changes, and osteoradionecrosis.[2] These complications negatively affect the patient's quality of life and ability to complete treatment. Effective oral care requires appropriate preventive and interceptive therapy,[3] patient and family education, and close observation. The maintenance of oral health during and after radiation therapy requires an investment of time and effort beyond that needed for normal oral care on the part of the patient and the practitioner.[4]

Acute Complications

Taste alteration (hypogeusia)

When the tongue is in the field of radiation, loss of sweet, salty, bitter, and acidic taste acuity can develop within the first weeks of therapy. The rate of loss is exponential as the dose accumulates to 3,000 cGy.[5] Taste acuity can be partially restored 20 to 60 days following completion of radiation. Residual hypogeusia can be seen in patients receiving greater then 6,000 cGy and may be exacerbated by xerostomia.

Mucositis

The onset, intensity, and duration of mucositis depends on the administered dose, dose fraction, type of ionizing radiation used, total dose given, the volume of tissue within the radiation portals, and continued use of tobacco and alcohol products.[6] Mucositis usually appears around 1,000 cGy at the beginning of the second week of treatment. It intensifies as treatment continues and resolves 2 or 3

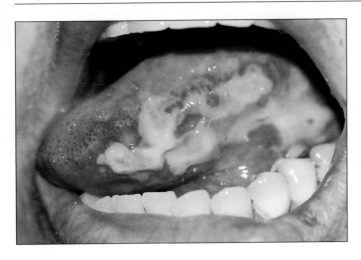

Fig 12-1 Severe oral mucositis secondary to radiation for squamous cell carcinoma of the lateral border of the tongue.

weeks after completion of therapy. The nonkeratinized tissues in the path of radiation (soft palate, pharynx, floor of the mouth, buccal mucosa, and base of tongue) are affected primarily and become erythematous and hyperemic. As the mucosa thins and atrophies due to decreased epithelial proliferation, small areas of denudation and ulceration covered with a white, fibrinous exudate occur (Fig 12-1). These areas may be focal at first, but can quickly become diffuse. Generalized sloughing can occur where the mucosal surfaces rub against each other, such as the lateral and ventral borders of the tongue or buccal mucosa[7] (Fig 12-2). Mucositis can be aggravated by mechanical irritation caused by faulty restorations, broken teeth, or ill-fitting prostheses (Figs 12-3 and 12-4). Patients with poor oral hygiene have an increased breakdown of inflamed marginal and interdental gingiva. Patients receiving dose-intensive treatment, such as a concomitant boost or implant, can have delayed healing.

Patients often experience pain and burning (even at rest) that is intensified by contact with coarse or spicy foods. They can also have difficulty swallowing or speaking. When symptoms are severe, treatment may be discontinued until the acute reactions subside.

Treatment of mucositis is mainly palliative, aimed at limiting tissue irritation, improving patient comfort, and controlling superinfection. A baking soda and salt water rinse (10 mL baking soda and 2.5 mL salt added to 0.95 L water) used four to six times a day facilitates pain relief, keeps oral tissues moist, and reduces oral debris. Good daily oral hygiene must be maintained with a soft brush and a bland-tasting dentifrice. This helps decrease the oral microflora and prevents infection. Use of broad spectrum antimicrobial rinses, such as chlorhexidine gluconate 0.12%, is effective in decreasing colonization of the oral flora, but is often poorly tolerated by the patient due to the high alcohol content. Studies conducted at several cancer centers showed that lozenges containing 2 g of polymyxin E, 1.8 mg of tobramycin, and 10 mg of amphotericin B may selectively eliminate gram-negative bacilli and yeast and prevent more severe mucositis.[8,9]

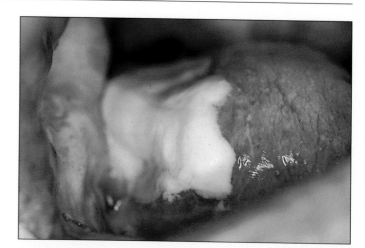

Fig 12-2 Soft tissue necrosis of the lateral border of the tongue, following radiation mucositis and mechanical trauma. The sharp edges of the lingual cusps can significantly increase a patient's discomfort. (Courtesy of Robert A. Ord.)

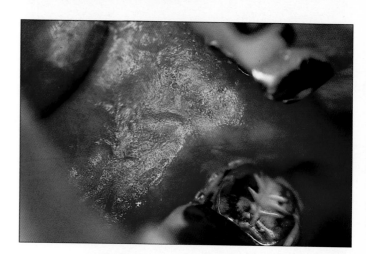

Fig 12-3 Radiation mucositis on the buccal mucosa adjacent to a gold crown.

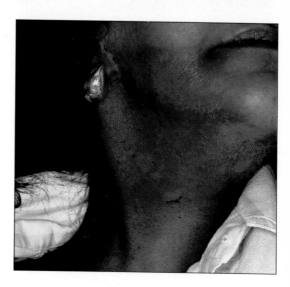

Fig 12-4 Erythema of the skin corresponding to the field of treatment in the patient in Fig 12-3.

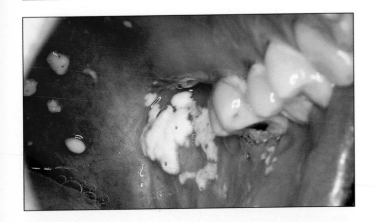

Fig 12-5 Pseudomembranous candidiasis in an irradiated patient.

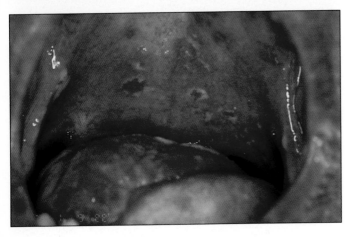

Fig 12-6 Severe erythema and candidiasis on the palate of a patient receiving radiation for tongue cancer. This patient also has angular cheilitis.

Sucralfate tablets, dissolved in water (1 g/15 mL) can be used as a rinsing agent for pain relief. It forms an adhesive paste that binds to ulcerated areas, creating a surface barrier.[10] Lidocaine (2%) or dyclonine hydrochloride (0.5%) can be combined with coating agents (magnesium hydroxide: Kaopectate, milk of magnesia) and diphenhydramine syrup (Benadryl elixir) to be used as a rinse and expectorant.[11-13] Kamillosan Liquidim solution (15 drops in 120 mL warm water), prepared from the flower of the chamomile plant, provides some reduction in inflammation and pain and may prevent severe mucositis.[14] Systemic analgesics can be important for pain control and allow for nutritional intake.

Infections

The most common infection is caused by *Candida albicans*. The infection is a result of decreased salivary flow and is exacerbated by dental prostheses and the continued use of alcohol and tobacco products.[15] In the pseudomembranous form, candidiasis appears as raised, white, cottage cheese–like plaques that can be scraped off, leaving an erythematous, bleeding base (Fig 12-5). In the atrophic or erythematous form, patchy reddened areas are found on the mucosa, particularly on the palate[16] (Fig 12-6). Patients often complain of a burning or stinging sensation. Topical antifungal agents (nystatin solution or clotrimazole troches) are the treatment of choice. For xerostomic patients, rinsing the mouth with water facilitates the dissolving of troches or tablets. Having the tissues cleansed of debris and prostheses removed allows maximum contact between the medication and oral tissues. Since acrylic denture bases often become colonized with *C albicans*, prostheses must be treated to prevent reinfection. Systemic infections rarely occur in patients receiving radiation because there is rarely significant immunosuppression.

Chronic Complications

Trismus

When the muscles of mastication and the temporomandibular joints are included in the radiation field,[16] such as in treatment of nasopharyngeal tumors, tumors of the retromolar pads, and posterior palate,[1] severe spasms may develop. Trismus can occur during treatment, but usually develops during the 6 months following treatment. Fibrosis of the muscles and the joint capsule can lead to limited mouth opening, which interferes with speech, mastication, and adequate oral hygiene. Trismus is usually more severe when radiation therapy is combined with surgical resection. Jaw exercises are essential preventive measures since the onset is gradual and often irreversible. Opening and closing the mouth as far as possible 20 times three times a day helps minimize muscle contracture and maintain normal function. Optimally, these exercises must continue for the first year and possibly longer.[17]

Once trismus develops, more aggressive physical therapy or prosthetic aids may be needed to regain lost interocclusal space. One method is the use of the maximum number of tongue blades that will fit passively between the incisal edges of the patient's mouth. Over time, additional blades are inserted into the middle of the stack to continuously increase the opening.[11] Mechanical versions, such as the Therabite Jaw Rehab System, can be used to stretch scar tissue and increase opening. However, once fibrosis has been established, physical therapy generally only limits further deterioration. Radical surgical procedures may be necessary to regain opening,[18] but can also lead to additional scarring and further decreased opening.

Xerostomia

The rapid onset of xerostomia is the most common side effect and a major source of morbidity in patients receiving radiation.[19] The severity and chronicity of the xerostomia is related to the dosage, radiation field, and amount of salivary tissue in the field.[20,21] Although salivary glands have relatively low mitotic rates, they are sensitive to radiation. The serous acini are the least radiation resistant, followed by the mucous cells and then the cells of the ductal system.[22] As a result, saliva becomes thick, tenacious, and viscous due to the higher loss of the serous component. Irreversible damage and hypofunction occurs at 4,000 cGy or higher. Patients receiving bilateral ionizing radiation involving the major salivary glands can show nearly an 80% decrease in stimulated and unstimulated flow compared to baseline measurements. Radiation of one parotid and one submandibular gland can produce up to a 60% reduction. Similarly, mantle radiation involving the lower border of the mandible affects salivary production of the sublingual and submandibular glands, resulting in measurable (72%) reduction in salivary production at rest.[23]

Patients report changes almost immediately, and studies have found up to a 50% reduction in salivary production following the first week of treatment (1,000 cGy) and greater than a 75% decline after 6 weeks (6,000 cGy).[6] Ongoing fibrosis can result in up to a 95% reduction in salivary flow 3 years after radiation.[16] Patients receiving radiation to the parotid glands, the major source of saliva during functional activities (eating and drinking), experience difficulty in eating dry foods, swallowing, and speaking. Patients who receive radiation to just the submandibular glands may report fewer changes during functional activities but increased difficulty at night.

In addition to a marked increase in viscosity and decrease in volume, there is a decrease in salivary pH to 5.5 and lower[24] with a concurrent loss in buffering capacity, decreases in electrolytes and immunoglobulin levels, and a shift in the oral microflora toward more cariogenic pathogens. Patients complain of burning sensations, discomfort, difficulty swallowing dry foods, and problems with food sticking to the teeth and mucosa.[25] There is decreased tolerance for spicy foods and increased sensitivity of the teeth to hot and cold. Candidal overgrowth is prevalent and the tongue can become atrophied and fissured. Inflammation and atrophy are common (Fig 12-7). As the mucosa becomes friable, ulcerations occur more frequently secondary to mechanical trauma (Fig 12-8). Patients have a low tolerance for dental prostheses because of this friability and lack of lubrication.[26]

Treatment is aimed at providing symptomatic relief. The use of salivary substitutes such as water, glycerin, and artificial saliva are frequently used. Carboxymethylcellulose and hydroxyethylcellulose preparations (Salivart, Oralube, Xerolube), mucopolysaccharide solutions (MouthKote), or glycerate polymer (OralBalance) help with moisture replacement and lubrication. Water mixed with glycerin can be used in a small spray bottle to keep mucosal tissues moist. Rinsing with a bland solution also helps moisturize tissues and aids in clearing mucus and debris. Commercial mouthrinses containing alcohol and/or phenol are not recommended because they can desiccate tissues further. Patients must be encouraged to drink more liquids to maintain sufficient hydration, take frequent sips of water during meals to help with swallowing, thin foods with liquids or gravies, and refrain from smoking and drinking alcohol or caffeine because of their drying effect. Humidifiers can be used at night to help with sleep-induced xerostomia.[19,27,28] Chewing sugarless gum or sucking on sugarless hard candies can help patients who have some residual salivary function.

Sialagogues that pharmacologically stimulate saliva production from responsive salivary gland tissue have shown some success. The most widely used products are pilocarpine hydrochloride (Salagen) and bethanechol. Pilocarpine stimulates salivary tissue by its muscarinic-cholinergic agonist properties.[29] Use of pilocarpine during radiation appears to significantly preserve salivary production. A therapeutic regimen of 5 mg four times a day is initiated just prior to radiation treatment and titrated to optimize clinical response and minimize adverse reactions. The common adverse side effects of sweating, rhinitis, headache, and urinary frequency are usually well tolerated.[30] The patient's bedtime dose can be increased to 10 mg after 1 week of starting the drug. If this is tolerated, the morning dose can be increased to a maximum of 10 mg. Increased salivary flow is usually seen within 30 minutes of ingestion, with maximal response only seen with continual use.[31] Pilocarpine is not recommended in patients with hypertension, cardiovascular disease, narrow angle glaucoma, or uncontrolled asthma.[32]

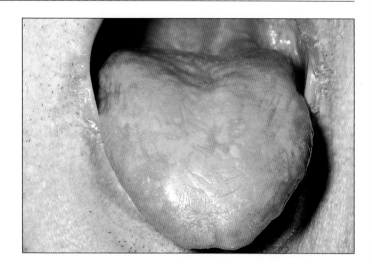

Fig 12-7 Tongue with atrophy of the papillae, inflammation, and denudation resulting from xerostomia.

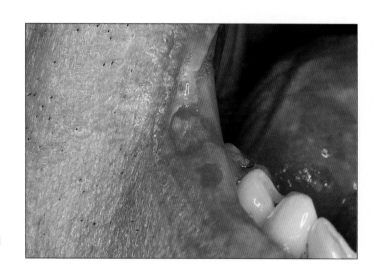

Fig 12-8 Ulceration of the labial mucosa secondary to radiation.

Bethanechol, a carbamic esther of beta-methycholine, has muscarinic and nicotinic cholinergic activity and can produce an increase in salivary production. Doses start at 25 mg three times daily and can be titrated up to 50 mg three times a day.[33]

Radiation Caries

Radiation does not directly cause dental caries. Xerostomia, resulting in decreased salivary pH, loss of buffering capacity, elimination of mechanical flushing of debris by saliva, loss of protective immunoproteins, and a shift in oral microflora toward more cariogenic species, contributes to rapid and devastating caries formation.[34] Destruction of salivary electrolytes (especially calcium and fluoride) decreases remineralization of tooth structure following acidic exposure. Radiation caries usually begins on the cervical surfaces, often leading to circumferential caries at the cementoenamel junction and amputation of crowns of the teeth within weeks or months[1] (Figs 12-9 to 12-11). Caries also form at the incisal edges and cusp tips in areas of previous attrition. Due to decreased vascularity and atrophy of pulpal tissues, patients have a decreased pain response[35] and often do not seek treatment until teeth are nonrestorable.

Radiation caries can be prevented by meticulous oral hygiene and daily application of topical fluoride. Neutral pH 1.1% sodium fluoride or 0.4% stannous fluoride gel can be used in a custom-fabricated carrier for 5 to 10 minutes a day.[36] The carrier must completely cover the teeth and extend several millimeters onto the marginal gingiva. Although stannous fluoride has greater penetration into tooth structure because of its acidic nature, it can cause pain and sensitivity in the teeth.[37] Some practitioners advocate combining fluoride with chlorhexidine in the same tray to help reduce the *Streptococcus mutans* level and increase remineralization.[38] In patients with a lesser degree of xerostomia, fluoride gel can be brushed on. Fluoride must be used daily because it leaches out of the tooth within 24 hours. It is vital that patients understand that fluoride must be used regularly for the rest of their lives and that radiation caries is not related to the radiation of the teeth, but rather is a result of irreversible xerostomia and a permanently changed oral environment.

Osteoradionecrosis

Osteoradionecrosis (ORN) is the most serious complication of radiation therapy. The cytotoxic effects of radiation on bone-forming cells, soft tissue fibrosis, and obliterative endarteritis result in hypoxic, hypocellular, and hypovascular bone and soft tissues.[39] This leaves these tissues with a diminished capacity for repair. Osteoradionecrosis is more likely to occur in the mandible than the maxilla. The greater density of bone absorbs more radiation, and the mandible's blood supply is limited and lacks the collateral circulation found in the maxilla. The incidence of ORN is proportional to the total dose delivered and is uncommon in patients receiving less than 6,000 cGy.[40] Use of both external beam therapy and intraoral implants increases the risk of ORN. Osteoradionecrosis often occurs when the mucosa is traumatized by tooth extraction, infection, aggressive periodontal treatment, or mechanical irritation (unopposed, supererupted teeth or dental prostheses), leading to exposure of the underlying bone.[13] Large areas of exposed, irregular bone can cause irritation and further breakdown of adjacent soft tissue (Figs 12-12 and 12-13). Patients may experience intractable pain, trismus, exfoliation of bony segments, and suppuration with the formation of extraoral and intraoral fistula. They

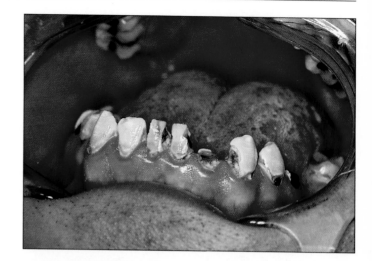

Fig 12-9 Radiation caries in a patient treated for Hodgkin's lymphoma who was noncompliant with fluoride use.

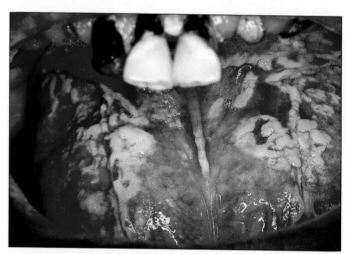

Fig 12-10 Circumferential caries with crown amputation postradiation. Pseudomembranous candidiasis is also present.

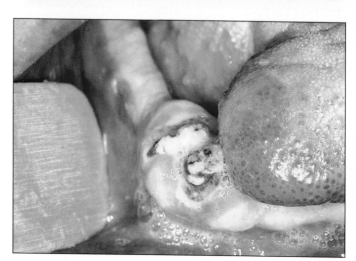

Fig 12-11 Radiation caries following radiation for a base of the tongue squamous cell carcinoma.

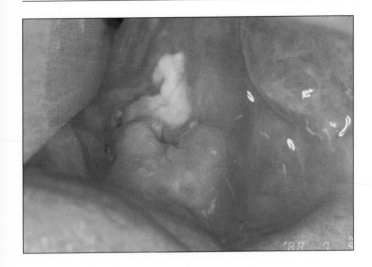

Fig 12-12 Area of osteoradionecrosis.

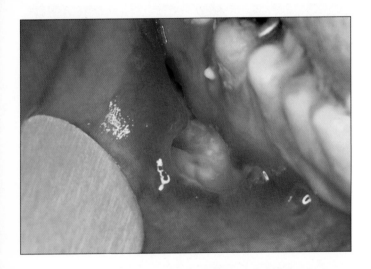

Fig 12-13 Area of soft tissue breakdown with exposure of necrotic bone.

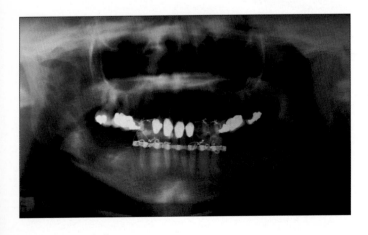

Fig 12-14 Bilateral ORN with pathologic fracture of the right mandible. (Courtesy of Robert A. Ord.)

may have difficulty eating, swallowing, or speaking. As the process progresses, pathologic fracture may occur (Fig 12-14).

Risk factors for the development of ORN include continued abuse of mucosal irritants such as alcohol and tobacco, poor oral hygiene, and compromised physical and nutritional status.[6] Extraction of teeth after radiation therapy is probably the highest risk factor for the development of ORN, making pretreatment evaluation critical. Grossly carious and periodontally involved teeth within the radiation ports should be extracted at least 14 days prior to initiation of therapy. Good primary closure is necessary to ensure adequate healing and prevent exposure of bone. In addition, all restorative care is best completed at this time. When ORN develops, a gentle, thorough debridement and irrigation, removal of sequestrum, and topical and systemic antimicrobial agents help promote healing. Use of hyperbaric oxygen helps promote osteoblast activity and healing for large exposed areas that do not respond to other treatments.[41] Hyperbaric oxygen can also be used prophylactically for postradiation extractions of mandibular teeth that were directly in the radiation field, especially in those patients who received radiation doses exceeding 6,000 cGy. Surgical resection is the last resort for treatment because of the possibility of further necrosis, physical disfigurement, and severe impairment in speech, chewing, and swallowing in an already debilitated patient.[42]

Oral Care Prior to Radiation

Every patient about to receive radiation to the head and neck must undergo a comprehensive dental evaluation to identify risk factors for the development of oral complications. All services required for the patient to be in optimal oral health need to be provided as well as initiation of an aggressive preventive regimen. Many patients with head and neck cancer are noncompliant with routine oral hygiene and dental care. Ninety-seven percent of dentulous patients need dental care prior to initiation of radiation.[43] Evaluation should be done at least 3 weeks before radiation to allow adequate time for wound healing. Knowledge of the location of the radiation field and total dose of radiation are important factors in formulating a treatment plan. For example, treatment of nasopharyngeal and soft palate tumors present a decreased risk for ORN since the body of the mandible is generally not in the field. Therefore, it is less critical to remove mandibular molars prior to initiation of radiation. For lesions in the floor of the mouth, tongue, and tonsillar pillar, and retromolar tumors that require radiation of the major salivary glands and the body of the mandible,[1] there is an increased risk of radiation caries and ORN. Practitioners need to be more aggressive about removal of questionable mandibular molars and premolars prior to radiation. If, due to the size or location of the primary tumor, the goal of radiation is palliation, preradiation extractions may only be indicated when retention of teeth could cause discomfort.[1]

A thorough oral examination should be performed, including:

- Full-mouth radiographs and a panoramic radiograph
- Identification of periodontal disease
- Bleeding index
- Pocket depths
- Tooth mobility
- Assessment of oral hygiene
- Assessment of the patient's motivation to comply with the necessary preventive regimen
- Identification of all restorative needs

- Carious lesions
- Defective restorations
- Fractured teeth
- Identification of periapical infections, unerupted teeth, root tips, and other pathologic conditions
- Preprosthetic surgical needs
- Bony ostosis
- Tori
- Evaluation of prosthetic appliances
- Proper fit and comfort
- Potential sources of irritation
- Removal of soft liners, which become colonized with yeast and can become a source of irritation to friable mucosa[44]

All teeth with a questionable prognosis, especially those in the radiation field, should be extracted prior to radiation. These include teeth with advanced caries, periapical pathosis, residual root tips, moderate to severe periodontal disease, impacted teeth not covered with bone, and unopposed teeth that may hypererupt and cause soft tissue trauma.[45] Aggressive care, especially extractions, should also be performed in patients with poor oral hygiene and little motivation or physical capacity to improve their oral status.[27,46] Extractions should be performed at least 2 to 3 weeks before radiation therapy begins to allow for complete mucosal healing. Coordination with the head and neck surgeon to perform extractions while the patient is receiving general anesthesia for oncologic surgical procedures prior to radiation is desirable, since this allows for adequate healing time. Alveolectomies are necessary to eliminate sharp ridges and bony spicules and to allow for primary closure. Any preprosthetic surgery (removal of tori or bony undercuts) should also be performed prior to radiation.

Scaling, root planing, and subgingival curettage to remove all hard and soft deposits should be performed. Any rough or sharp tooth surfaces or restorations should be smoothed or replaced. Carious teeth need to be restored. Nonvital teeth that are important for function and are not in the primary beam or a high-risk area of the mandible can be treated endodontically.[2] Mandibular molars with periapical pathosis in the field should be extracted due to a higher rate of failed endodontics associated with multirooted teeth and a risk of ORN.

Patients and their families must be aware of the side effects of radiation and the implications associated with neglect. Explicit oral hygiene instructions are vitally important and must be reiterated frequently. Patients unable to maintain a healthy dental status are best served by having all remaining teeth extracted. The importance of daily plaque removal using a soft toothbrush, floss, interproximal brushes, and fluoridated dentifrice needs to be stressed.

Fabrication of custom fluoride applicators and initiation of daily fluoride use should be started immediately. It is imperative that patients understand that they must use the fluoride indefinitely to prevent the development of radiation caries and that fluoride alone is not a substitute for good oral hygiene.[47] Patients must realize that radiation caries can develop years after radiation therapy and that fluoride and aggressive oral hygiene are a lifelong necessity.[46]

In patients who have trouble with adequate nutritional intake, high-sugar foods and liquids are often recommended to increase calories. To decrease caries risk, patients should brush immediately after eating.[48] Following the completion of radiation, dietary counseling to help patients avoid food items that cause prolonged sugar exposure can help prevent caries formation.

Oral Care During Radiation Therapy

During radiation, patients need to be monitored weekly. Palliative treatment of mucositis includes frequent salt–baking soda rinses to reduce mucosal irritation and remove secretions and debris. Dilute chlorhexidine rinses three to four times a day can be used as tolerated to decrease gingival inflammation. Rinses made with diphenhydramine, kaolin with pectin, and topical anesthetics can provide topical pain relief. Specimens of any severe areas of tissue necrosis and/or mucositis that develop outside the radiation field should be cultured to rule out viral or bacterial infection.[49] Patients should also be checked for candidal infection.

Use of saliva substitutes should be encouraged to lubricate dried mucosal tissues and decrease the chance of traumatic ulceration. Patients can be started on a diet of semisoft food, moistened with liquids or gravies, and cautioned to avoid spicy, acidic, or mechanically irritating foods. Good oral hygiene and daily fluoride use must be reinforced.

Trismus prevention exercises should be reviewed. If measurement of the interarch distance shows decreased opening, the exercise program can be intensified or a mechanical device prescribed. Denture wearing should be discouraged, except for obturators. Necessary restorative work on teeth outside of the primary beam can be continued as long as patients can tolerate treatment.

Oral Care After Radiation Therapy

Following the completion of radiation therapy, patients should be observed once or twice during the first month. Then they can be placed on a 3- to 4-month recall schedule. The goal is to prevent radiation caries and periodontal disease, decrease the risk of development of ORN, and manage some of the chronic side effects, such as xerostomia. Questions about the severity of xerostomia and any subjective complaints should be correlated with clinical assessment of the degree of hyposalivation, appearance of the oral mucosa, level of salivary secretion, and composition and viscosity of saliva. The oral mucosa should be examined for areas of irritation or ulceration. If present, the causative agent should be identified and corrected if possible. Adherence to oral hygiene and fluoride protocol needs to be reinforced.

The interarch distance should be measured at follow-up to determine if there is decreased oral opening. Trismus can develop up to 1 year after completion of radiation therapy. Patients should be encouraged to continue jaw opening exercises, and physiotherapy should be initiated if these exercises do not prevent trismus.

The dentition should be checked for calculus and areas of demineralization or caries. Pocket depths and bleeding indices can help indicate any change in the patient's periodontal health. Gentle scaling and root planing and polishing to remove hard and soft deposits can be performed. Teeth that were directly in the primary radiation beam have decreased capacity for repair and regeneration of the periodontium due to loss of vascularity in the periodontal ligament.[50] Reattachment after rigorous scaling and curettage or mucogingival surgery may not occur, creating periodontal pockets that can lead to infection and bone necrosis. Therefore, decreased tissue tolerance and healing capacity must be considered prior to initiating aggressive periodontal therapy.

Carious lesions and areas of demineralization need to be treated immediately, due to rapid progression. Patients rarely present with isolated areas of decay. Lesions must be thoroughly excavated. Placement of a fluoride-releasing liner or base may help with recurrent decay at the margins. Due to the altered oral environment and xerostomia, resin-bonded restorations may need to be replaced more frequently.[44] Amalgam should be used in cases in which a good etch cannot be achieved or the lesion extends either subgingivally or into difficult to reach interproximal and root areas.[1] Large circumferential lesions may need to be restored in stages. Once radiation caries develops, recurrent decay around recently placed restorations is common. In teeth that are not restorable, endodontic therapy can be performed without increased risk of ORN[35] and coronal amputation can be performed rather than extraction.

Because trauma to the alveolar ridge by prosthetic appliances can precipitate ORN, the timing of prosthetic rehabilitation is one of considerable debate. The decision must be based on clinical judgment and the condition of the mucosa. Patients who are edentulous and wore dentures prior to radiation are at significantly lower risk of developing ORN than patients who undergo preradiation or postradiation extractions.[41] For those completely recovered from their mucositis who have well-fitting dentures, relining the existing prosthesis may be possible 3 months following the completion of radiation. For patients with a prolonged mucositis, significant xerostomia with atrophied, friable mucosa, or recent extractions in the field of radiation, the waiting time before considering prosthetic rehabilitation can be 6 months to a year.[51] In noncompliant patients who are at risk, the decision may be made not to fabricate dentures at all. Care must be taken that there is no overextension of the borders, that areas of scar tissue are adequately relieved, and that lateral movements of the mandibular base are minimized by careful occlusal adjustment. Proper denture hygiene should be stressed and patients instructed to remove the dentures at night. Frequent postinsertion checks are extremely important to prevent mucosal perforation with bone exposure, especially in the mylohyoid and retromylohyoid areas. Patients should remove the prosthesis at the first sign of irritation and be examined by their dentist immediately.

Postradiation extractions are a significant cause of ORN.[52-54] There is little agreement among investigators about the relationship between the time elapsed from completion of radiation therapy to tooth removal and the occurrence of ORN.[55] Extractions must be performed with careful handling of the soft tissue, alveolectomies, primary wound closure, and antibiotic coverage. In irradiated patients at high risk of developing ORN (those with compromised blood supply secondary to surgery, receiving greater than 6,000 cGy to mandibular segments, with poor mucosal integrity, or in generally poor physical condition), the use of multiple sessions of hyperbaric oxygen preoperatively and postsurgically is recommended.[56] Alternative treatment to extraction is endodontic therapy with crown amputation.

Summary

The primary goal in the treatment of patients receiving head and neck radiation is prevention and management of oral complications. Since the potential for significant morbidity exists, prompt, effective oral management is essential and requires collaboration by the dentist, oncologist, and other oncologic specialists. Awareness of the acute and chronic complications of radiation therapy can help the dentist reduce or prevent serious sequelae and improve the patient's outcome.

References

1. Carl W. Oral and dental care of patients receiving radiation therapy for tumors in and around the oral cavity. In: Carl W, Sako K (eds). Cancer and the Oral Cavity, ed 1. Chicago: Quintessence, 1986;167–182.

2. Beumer J, Curtis T, Harrison RE. Radiation therapy of the oral cavity: Sequelae and management. Part 1. Head Neck Surg 1979;1:301–312.

3. Semba SE, Mealey B, Hallman WW. The head and neck radiotherapy patient. Part I. Oral manifestations of radiation therapy. Compend Contin Educ Dent 1992;15:250–260.

4. Carl W. Local radiation and systemic chemotherapy: Preventing and managing the oral complications. J Am Dent Assoc 1993;124:119–123.

5. National Institutes of Health Consensus Development Conference on Oral Complications of Cancer Therapies: Diagnosis, prevention and treatment. NCI Monogr 1990;9:3–8.

6. Dreizen S. Description and incidence of oral complications. NCI Monogr 1990;9:11–15.

7. Toth BB, Chambers MS, Fleming TC. Prevention and management of oral complications associated with cancer therapies: Radiotherapy/chemotherapy. Tex Dent J 1996;113:23–29.

8. Spijkervat FKL, van Saene HKF, van Saene JJM, Panders AK, Vermey A, Mehta DM. Effects of selective elimination of oral flora on mucositis in irradiated head and neck cancer patients. J Surg Oncol 1991; 46:167–173.

9. Symonds B. Treatment induced mucositis: An old problem with new remedies. Br J Cancer 1998;77: 1689–1695.

10. Barker G, Loftus L, Cuddy P, Baker B. The effects of sucralfate suspension and diphenhydramine syrup plus kaolin pectin on radiotherapy induced mucositis. Oral Surg Oral Med Oral Pathol 1991;71:288–293.

11. Whitmyer C, Waskowski J, Iffland H. Radiotherapy and oral sequelae: Prevention and management protocols. J Dent Hyg 1997;71:23–29.

12. Scully C, Epstein JB. Oral health care for the cancer patient. Eur J Cancer B Oral Oncol 1996;32B: 281–292.

13. Fleming TJ. Oral tissue changes in radiation oncology and their management. Dent Clin North Am 1990;34:223–237.

14. Carl W, Emrich L. Management of oral mucositis during local radiation and systemic chemotherapy: A study of 98 patients. J Prosthet Dent 1991;66: 361–369.

15. Epstein JB, Marshall M, Le ND, et al. Risk factors for candidiasis in patients who receive radiation therapy for malignant conditions of the head and neck. Oral Surg Oral Med Oral Pathol 1993;76:169–174.

16. Dreizen S, Daly TE, Drane JB, et al. Oral complications of cancer radiotherapy. Postgrad Med 1977;61:85–92.

17. Barret VJ, Martin JW, Jacob RF. Physical therapy techniques in treatment of head and neck patients. J Prosthet Dent 1988;59:343–346.

18. McClure D, Barker G, Barker B. Oral management of the cancer patient, Part II: Oral complications of radiation therapy. Compend Contin Educ Dent 1987;8: 88–92.

19. Garg AK, Malo M. Manifestations and treatment of xerostomia and associated oral effects secondary to head and neck radiation therapy. J Am Dent Assoc 1997;128:1128–1133.

20. Markitziu A, Zafiropoulous G, Tsalik L. Gingival health and salivary function in head and neck irradiated patients. Oral Surg Oral Med Oral Pathol 1992; 73:427–433.

21. Valdez H. Radiation-induced salivary gland dysfunction: Clinical course and significance. Spec Care Dentist 1991;11:252–255.

22. Stephens LC, Schylthesis TE, Price RE. Radiation apoptosis of serous acinar cells of salivary glands. Cancer 1991;67:1539–1543.

23. Liu RP, Fleming TJ, Toth BB. Salivary flow rates in patients with head and neck cancer, 5–25 years after radiation. Oral Surg Oral Med Oral Pathol 1990;70:724–729.

24. Carl W. Oral complications of local and systemic cancer treatment. Curr Opin Oncol 1995;7:320–324.

25. Atkinson JC, Wu AS. Salivary gland dysfunction: Causes, symptoms, treatment. J Am Dent Assoc 1994; 125:409–416.

26. Guchelaar HS, Vermes A, Meerwaldt JH. Radiation-induced xerostomia: Pathophysiology, clinical course and supportive treatment. Support Care Cancer 1997;5:281–288.

27. Reynolds WR, Hickey AJ, Feldman MI. Dental management of the cancer patient receiving radiation therapy. Clin Prev Dent 1980;2:5–9.

28. McClure D, Barker G, Barker B. Oral complications of head and neck radiation therapy. In: Barker B. Oral Management of the Cancer Patient. Kansas City: University of Missouri-Kansas City School of Dentistry, 1989:1–13.

29. Fox PC, VanderVen PF, Baum BJ, Mandel D. Pilocarpine for xerostomia associated with salivary gland dysfunction. Oral Surg Oral Med Oral Pathol 1986;61:243–245.

30. Greenspan D. Management of salivary gland dysfunction. NCI Monogr 1990;9:159–161.

31. Valdez IH, Wolff A, Atkinson JC, Macynski AA, Fox PC. Use of pilocarpine during head and neck radiation therapy to reduce xerostomia and salivary gland dysfunction. Cancer 1993;71:1848–1851.

32. Johnson JT, Ferretti GA, Nethery WJ. Oral pilocarpine for postradiation xerostomia in patients with head and neck radiation. N Engl J Med 1993;329:390–395.

33. Epstein JB, Burchcell JC, Emerton S, Le ND, Silverman S. A clinical trial of bethanechol in patients with xerostomia after radiation therapy. Oral Surg Oral Med Oral Pathol 1994;77:610–614.

34. Brown LR, Dreizin SA, Daly TE. Interrelations of oral microorganisms, immunoglobulins and dental caries following radiotherapy. J Dent Res 1978;57:882–893.

35. Seto BG, Beumer J, Kagawa T. Analysis of endodontic therapy in patients irradiated for head and neck cancer. Oral Surg Oral Med Oral Pathol 1985; 60:540–545.

36. Dreizen S, Brown LR, Daly TE, Drane JB. Prevention of xerostomia related dental caries in irradiated cancer patients. J Dent Res 1977;56:99–104.

37. Toth BB, Chambers MS, Fleming TJ, Lemon JC, Martin JW. Minimizing oral complications of cancer treatment. Oncology 1995;9:851–858.

38. Katz S. The use of fluoride and chlorhexidine for the prevention of radiation caries. J Am Dent Assoc 1982;104:164–170.

39. Marx RE. Osteoradionecrosis: A new concept of its pathophysiology. J Oral Maxillofac Surg 1988;41:283–288.

40. Beumer J, Silverman S Jr, Benak SB Jr. Hard and soft tissue necrosis following radiation therapy for oral cancer. J Prosthet Dent 1972;27:640–644.

41. Friedman R. Osteoradionecrosis: Causes and prevention. NCI Monogr 1990;9:145–149.

42. Barker B. Oral complications of head and neck radiation. Compend Contin Educ Dent 1987;8:288–293.

43. Lockhart PB, Clark S. Pretherapy dental status of patients with malignant conditions of the head and neck. Oral Surg Oral Med Oral Pathol 1994; 77:236–241.

44. Jansma J, Vissink A, Spijkervet F, et al. Protocol for the prevention and treatment of oral sequelae resulting from head and neck radiation therapy. Cancer 1992;70:2171–2180.

45. Beumer J, Harrison R, Sandlers B, Kurrasch M. Osteoradionecrosis: Predisposing factors and outcomes of therapy. Head Neck Surg 1984;6:819–827.

46. Nguyen AMH. Dental management of patients who receive chemo- and radiation therapy. Gen Dent 1992;40:305–311.

47. Epstein JB, Vandermeij EH, Lunn R, Le ND, Stevenson-Moore P. Effects of compliance with fluoride gel on caries and caries risk in patients after radiation therapy for head and neck cancer. Oral Surg Oral Med Oral Pathol 1996;82:268–274.

48. Minasian A, Dwyer J. Nutritional implications of dental and swallowing issues in head and neck cancer. Oncology 1998;12:1155–1161.

49. Epstein JB, Vandermeij EH. Complicating mucosal reactions in patients receiving radiation therapy for head and neck cancer. Spec Care Dentist 1997;17:89–93.

50. Silverman S, Chieria G. Radiation therapy of oral carcinoma I: Effects on the oral tissues and management of the periodontium. J Periodontol 1965;36:478–484.

51. Beumer J, Curtis T, Marrish R. Radiation complications in edentulous patients. J Prosthet Dent 1976;36:193–203.

52. Beumer J, Curtis T, Harrison RE. Radiation therapy of the oral cavity: Sequelae and management. Part 2. Head Neck Surg 1979;1:392–408.

53. Beumer J, Harrison R, Sanders B, et al. Postradiation dental extractions: A review of the literature and a report of 72 episodes. Head Neck Surg 1983;6:581–586.

54. Murray CG, Herson J, Daly TE, et al. Radiation necrosis of the mandible: A 10 year study. Part II. Dental factors, onset, duration and management of necrosis. Int J Radiat Oncol Biol Phys 1980;6:549–553.

55. Starke EN, Shanon I. How critical is the interval between extractions and irradiation in patients with head and neck malignancy? J Oral Surg 1997;43:333–337.

56. Marx RE, Johnson RP, Kline SN. Prevention of osteoradionecrosis: A randomized prospective clinical trial of hyperbaric oxygen vs penicillin. J Am Dent Assoc 1985;111:49–54.

CHAPTER 13

Surgical Treatment of the Patient Receiving Radiation Therapy

Remy H. Blanchaert, Jr, MD, DDS

Radiation therapy has a well-established role in the management of carcinoma of the oral cavity. Radiation therapy is used as a sole treatment modality in early stage (stage I and stage II) disease. In late stage disease, radiation therapy is typically administered following surgical resection (adjuvant radiation therapy) or in conjunction with chemotherapy (organ preservation protocols). Radiation causes cellular injury in a dose-dependent fashion. Tumor cells are more susceptible to radiation than normal tissues. Normal cells also recover from radiation therapy more quickly. Therapy is therefore delivered in a particular time and dose fashion to maximize tumor cell kill while limiting normal cell injury.

For the purposes of surgical decision making, this chapter is divided into two sections based on timing of surgery in relation to radiation therapy. The first portion of the chapter deals with the surgical principles involved in the care of patients prior to or during radiation therapy and focuses on limiting the delay of therapy and complications. The second section explores the treatment of the surgical patient after receiving radiation therapy and focuses on the difficulties of late reconstruction and the management of osteoradionecrosis. It must always be remembered that the effects of radiation therapy are permanent and progressive. The surgeon must always respect the tissue injury and impairment of the natural healing process inherent in the delivery of radiation therapy. Communication between the dentist, surgeon, and radiation therapist is mandatory if complications are to be avoided or minimized.

Surgical Management of Patients Prior to Radiation Therapy

Surgical intervention prior to radiation therapy is common. The majority of patients with advanced stage (stage III and stage IV) tumors undergo resection prior to radiation therapy. Radiation therapy is administered in these cases because there is documented improvement in disease-free survival for such patients. Patients with advanced primary cancers, close surgical resection margins, bone invasion by tumor, perineural and lymphatic invasion, or extracapsular extension of disease benefit from adjuvant radiation therapy.

The modern goal of surgery is to achieve a one-stage resection of the disease process (primary tumor and draining lymphatics) and definitive reconstruction. Increasingly, the use of free tissue transfer has made these goals a reality. In the past, patients often underwent resection and radiation therapy prior to definitive reconstruction. The scarring and fibrosis resulting from such treatment was almost impossible to overcome secondarily. The proponents of such therapy contend that in this manner only those patients likely to survive the disease undergo reconstruction. Modern thought contends that all patients should receive definitive treatment in one setting. Those patients unlikely to survive should undergo primary reconstruction because of the improvement in quality of life (intelligible speech, oral swallowing, decannulation from tracheostomy). Likewise, a return to the hospital for additional surgery impacts negatively on quality of life.

Many patients with oral cancers that require radiation therapy are dentate. Professional management of the dentition is mandatory prior to radiation therapy. A dental consultation prior to radiation therapy warrants immediate, direct attention. In many cases there has been a delay in diagnosis, leading to further delay of therapy, which allows for tumor progression. Dental consultations should be handled urgently. Definitive treatment plans should be developed and therapy carried out as soon as possible. On occasion dental surgical procedures are carried out at the time of ablative cancer surgery.

For the purposes of this chapter, preradiation surgical management is separated into

issues concerning dentoalveolar surgery and management of the mandible in access osteotomies.

Dentoalveolar surgery

Preparation of the patient with oral cancer for the rigors of radiation therapy requires the dentist or oral surgeon to understand the particulars of the planned treatment. Radiation therapy typically requires radiation doses above 50 Gy, which place the oral soft tissues and bone at risk for osteoradionecrosis. The severity of the complications that develop in mismanaged cases warrant strict adherence to dental management protocols. Full dental evaluation requires physical examination, radiography, and discussion with the patient. Carious or periodontally involved teeth and partial impactions (not full bony impactions without pathosis) are extracted. Bone exostoses and mandibular tori are removed. Surgery is best performed at least 2 weeks prior to the initiation of radiation therapy. There is a marked decrease in the risk of osteoradionecrosis if the surgical sites have some time to heal prior to radiation.[1] Maxillary tori are removed only if large and at significant risk due to recurring trauma.

Osteoradionecrosis is a complication of therapy that develops when injury occurs to the soft tissues overlying irradiated bone or when dental extraction is required and the native tissues lack sufficient reserve to heal the injury. Common sites for the development of osteoradionecrosis are the mandibular alveolar ridge, mandibular tori, and the mylohyoid line (Fig 13-1). Osteoradionecrosis is discussed at length in the next section of this chapter.

An understanding of the patient's motivation and oral hygiene skills is required to make appropriate decisions regarding dental extrac-

Fig 13-1 (a) Dental extractions following radiation therapy resulted in chronic exposure of alveolar bone. (b) Osteoradionecrosis resulted in pathologic fracture and bone extrusion.

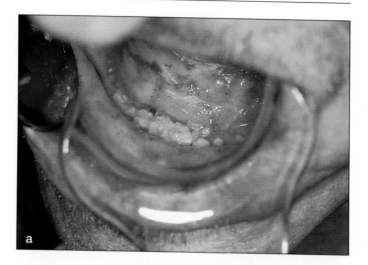

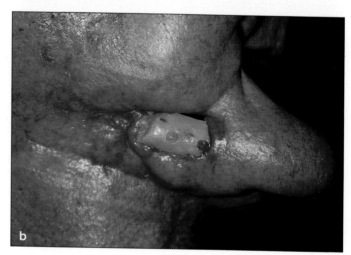

tions. Whenever a question exists about patient willingness or ability to comply with the necessary home care routine for maintenance of the dentition, full-mouth extraction is completed. In carefully selected patients, the maintenance of an intact dentition positively impacts the outcome following therapy. An incorrect decision, however, places both the patient and the dentist in a very difficult position.

At the University of Maryland, all patients are evaluated initially by general dentistry and oral and maxillofacial surgery residents before radiation therapy, then presented to one of two providers who make the final decisions regarding necessary dental therapy. These practitioners (one general dentist, one oral surgeon) collaborate in the development of a standard protocol in decision making, documentation, and therapy. This facilitates timeliness of care delivery, continuity of care, and resident education. Oral hygiene instruction, fluoride tray fabrication, and care are delivered by a single dental hygienist, whose input into the patient's motivation is particularly helpful.

Mandibular surgery

Collaboration between the ablative and reconstructive surgical teams is necessary to allow full utilization of the complementary skills of these two disciplines, and an important consideration is the restoration of mandibular continuity. In the case of composite resection, it is preferable that the mandible is reconstructed primarily with a microvascular free tissue transfer, although on occasion stabilization with a rigid reconstruction bar alone is necessary. In some tumors, visualization of the margins of the tumor is enhanced by mandibulotomy techniques. Careful performance and stabilization of the mandibulotomy are critical to early bone healing prior to initiation of radiation therapy. Locating the mandibulotomy in the symphysis region is ideal because it often places the osteotomy outside the field of the radiation injury (mandibulotomies are typically carried out for tongue base and lateral pharynx tumors). Some surgeons prefer rigid bicortical stabilization. Others use two monocortical semirigid plates. The majority of the literature supports selection of some form of rigid stabilization over nonrigid techniques. Numerous articles have documented decreased rates of infection, mobility, nonunion, and malocclusion with rigid techniques of mandibulotomy stabilization.[2,3]

Surgical Treatment of Patients After Radiation Therapy

Radiation therapy results in the development of a hypoxic, hypocellular, hypovascular tissue environment. The effect is such that there is limited capacity for the tissue involved to respond to injury with an appropriate neovascularization as seen in wound healing following injury to normal tissue. In normal (nonirradiated) tissue following wounding, a zone of hypoxia with a steep oxygen tension gradient develops between the center of the wounded area and the immediate surrounding tissues. This gradient cannot be created within a field of significant radiation injury because of the already low oxygen tension in the surrounding tissues. These factors must be taken into consideration by anyone planning elective surgery within a field of previous radiation where the dose was greater than 60 Gy. Clearly, manipulation of this environment to create a more normal tissue response is required. Hyperbaric oxygen therapy is the most common means by which these tissues can be altered favorably. It is useful because it allows the creation of oxygen tension gradients capable of inducing favorable responses following wounding within the irradiated tissue field.

Macrophages are the most important cellular element in wounded tissues because of the role they play in the initiation and control of complex mechanisms of tissue repair. The oxygen tension gradient produced in wounds acts as a chemoattractant to the macrophages. They therefore accumulate in the wound and are stimulated to secrete macrophage-derived angiogenesis factor (MDAF) and macrophage-derived growth factor (MDGF). These cytokines result in the induction of the formation of new blood vessels and the mitoses of mesenchymal cells and fibroblasts. These are certainly not the only cytokines active in wounds. Research has delineated an ever-expanding number of such mediators. It is possible to manipulate MDAF and MDGF to enhance the healing potential of irradiated tissues.

The role of oxygen gradients in wound healing has been well documented for years.

Excellent works by Hunt and Dai[4] and Knighton et al[5,6] explored this subject many years ago. Further work by Marx et al[7] defined the mechanism by which the administration of hyperbaric oxygen can produce an environment in irradiated tissue that mimics that occurring in normal injured tissues. Their work provided excellent documentation for and an explanation of a concept that had already been in widespread use for years. Likewise, they helped to delineate the absence of improved wound healing in nonirradiated tissue following hyperbaric oxygen administration. Clearly once a wound is able to overcome the severe oxygen tension gradient seen in irradiated tissue and approaches that of normal wounded tissue, the effects of hyperbaric oxygen therapy drop off sharply.

The following section deals with evidence-supported decision making in regard to the elective (secondary) reconstruction of patients following radiation therapy and the management of osteoradionecrosis. Particularly relevant to the following discussion is an understanding of the mechanism of action of hyperbaric oxygen therapy as previously outlined and its role in such cases.

Elective surgery in irradiated patients

Patients who have received radiation to 60 Gy or more are at significant risk for postoperative complications related to limitations in tissue healing response. The risk is lifelong and progressively greater as the time since radiation therapy increases. This concept was once ignored. Previous teaching held that as time progressed, the effects of radiation therapy were diminished. This has clearly been disproved.[1] Common situations in which patients require surgical procedures following radia-

tion therapy are dental extraction and secondary mandibular reconstruction. As previously mentioned, consideration for extractions prior to radiation should be mandatory; however, this is not always the case. Likewise, primary mandibular reconstruction with microvascular free tissue transfer (see chapter 8) is preferable to delayed reconstruction. The dentist and surgeon are frequently faced with treatment of such patients following radiation therapy. Thankfully, valuable contributions to scientific knowledge regarding hyperbaric medicine have allowed for manipulation of the unfavorable hypovascular, hypocellular, and hypoxic irradiated environment to a more favorable, better oxygenated environment.

A presurgical evaluation of patients for dental extraction should include the amount, type, and field of radiation delivered. The surgeon may find that the teeth in question were in fact spared from the primary radiation beam (eg, teeth in the mandibular symphysis following radiation therapy for larynx carcinoma). In this situation there is no contraindication to extraction or need for adjunctive hyperbaric oxygen therapy. Standard gentle surgical technique with minimal trauma and primary closure of the extraction site should result in appropriate healing in such patients.

Patients who have received radiation doses greater than 60 Gy to a site of planned extractions may benefit from presurgical hyperbaric oxygen. Marx et al[8] defined the standard protocol for this situation through a randomized controlled trial of hyperbaric oxygen versus antibiotic therapy. Twenty preoperative treatments and 10 treatments after surgery were selected as the standard based on experiments outlining the return of tissue oxygen gradients to near normal levels following 20 treatments. Each treatment involved inspiration of 100% oxygen via facemask while at 2.4 atm for 90 minutes. Hyperbaric oxygen was found to significantly decrease the risk of osteoradionecro-

169

sis following tooth extraction. Two groups of 37 patients each underwent extraction of 135 teeth (penicillin group) and 156 teeth (hyperbaric oxygen group). Osteoradionecrosis was seen in 11 (29.9%) of the antibiotic group and 2 (5.4%) of the hyperbaric oxygen group.

There is significant cost related to the administration of hyperbaric oxygen, as well as some limitations to access to a hyperbaric chamber. The costs of hyperbaric oxygen therapy vary among institutions, based mostly on size and use of the chamber. Occasionally, third-party agencies refuse to provide authorization for hyperbaric oxygen therapy. In such cases, the dentist or surgeon should provide copies of literature supporting hyperbaric oxygen therapy to both the insurance company's physician-reviewer and the patient. The article by Marx et al[8] is recommended, as it outlines costs directly.

The same protocol is used for elective secondary mandibular reconstructions in patients who have been selected for free bone grafting following radiation therapy. The author prefers to use free vascularized bone flaps in such cases; however, the skills of a microvascular surgeon may not be available in all locations. In this case, the author performs free tissue transfer and the standard protocol of hyperbaric oxygen is still used. The therapy enhances the vascularity of the residual mandible to which the flap will be attached, theoretically improving the rate of direct bone union. When free bone grafting is used, additional soft tissue flaps are often required to counteract the effect of scarring and the fibrosis present in the native irradiated tissues. This tissue (typically a pedicled muscle flap) has a significant impact on the blood supply and therefore the revascularization of the bone graft. Additional support for the rate of healing of the bone graft can be obtained through the use of platelet-rich plasma enhancement of the graft (Fig 13-2). Marx et al[9] described this technique in 1998. It is critical that the bone graft not be exposed to the bacteria present in the oral cavity or saliva. Contamination in such a strained wound environment commonly results in the development of an infection and loss of the bone graft.

Osteoradionecrosis

Surgeons and dentists involved in the care of patients with head and neck cancer encounter osteoradionecrosis at some point. Early wisdom held that nonhealing wounds of bone following radiation therapy were the result of infection.[10] A more modern theory proposed by Marx[11] in 1983 described a series of events leading to chronic painful exposure of bone that fails to heal in the face of radiation therapy. It detailed the sequential events leading to osteoradionecrosis as radiation, the development of a hypoxic-hypocellular-hypovascular tissue environment, soft tissue breakdown, and a chronic nonhealing wound.

Marx documented this triad (hypoxic, hypocellular, and hypovascular) by examining 26 cases of osteoradionecrosis. In his series, 17 of 26 patients had well-defined episodes of trauma following radiation injury. Fifteen of these events were tooth extraction and the other two were caused by denture trauma. The radiation doses of those without well-defined traumatic inciting factors were found to be especially high. Significant differences between osteoradionecrosis and osteomyelitis exist in regard to the type of bacteria seen and the nature of the bacterial insult. In the patients with osteoradionecrosis, only surface colonization of bone was seen; no deep invasion was identified. The type of colonization suggested that the bacteria and yeast were saprophytic contaminates. This differs markedly from osteomyelitis in infected bone grafts of the jaws in which invasion of the medullary space by organisms such as

Fig 13-2 (a,b) Secondary mandibular reconstruction with free bone grafting is to be undertaken in this case. Exposure of the mandibular defect has been accomplished. Note the degree of fibrosis within the irradiated field. (c-e) Autogenous cancellous marrow from the posterior ilium is combined with platelet-rich plasma as described by Marx et al.[9] (f,g) Coagulation of the platelet-rich plasma within the bone graft produces a firm moldable graft that can easily be placed within the existing defect. The growth factors elaborated by the platelets enhance the revascularization and maturation of the graft.

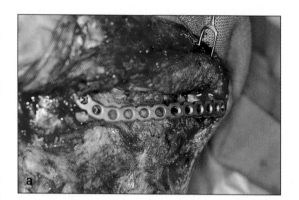

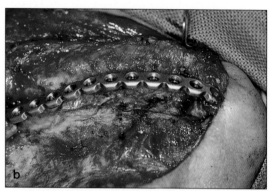

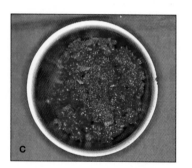

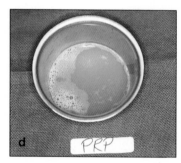

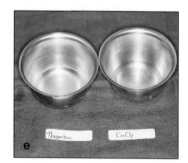

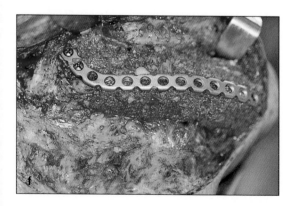

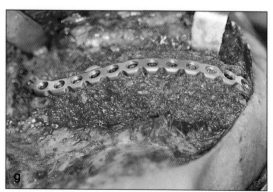

Bacteroides, *Eikenella*, and *Staphylococcus* are commonly seen. All of the patients in this study had received greater than 60 Gy of radiation.

Marx[12] described the cellular changes seen in radiation therapy that are important in the development of osteoradionecrosis. He reported the histologic findings of resection specimens from patients with osteoradionecrosis. He described endothelial cell death, hyalinization, and thrombosis of vessels. He reported that periosteum becomes fibrotic, osteoblasts and osteocytes die, and marrow spaces are filled with fibrous tissue. Mucosa and skin are less cellular and more fibrotic following radiation therapy. Decreased vascularity was seen in all connective tissue.

Surgeons and dentists are often called on to manage the poor dental health of patients with oral cancer prior to radiation therapy. Marx and Johnson[1] reported outcomes from four studies of a total database of 536 patients. Their report identified a specific period of risk for osteoradionecrosis. Three distinct patterns were seen across a timeline. In one group osteoradionecrosis developed as a result of the concomitant application of wounding and radiation therapy. In the second group, osteoradionecrosis developed spontaneously in relation to massive doses of radiation. In the third group osteoradionecrosis developed because of wounding distant to the application of radiation therapy and therefore in a field of hypovascular, hypocellular, hypoxic tissue.

By closely examining the group of patients in whom osteoradionecrosis developed in relation to concomitant injury and radiation therapy, a clear time factor was seen. The performance of extractions within 3 weeks of the initiation of radiation therapy was found to be a major risk factor. No cases of osteoradionecrosis were induced when 3 weeks of healing was allowed prior to radiation therapy.

The authors therefore recommended that, when possible, this 3-week period of healing should be respected.[1] This goal can often be accomplished if radiation therapy is not the sole treatment modality. Commonly, patients who are to undergo surgery need wound recovery times of 3 to 4 weeks before initiation of radiation therapy. Therefore extractions performed prior to surgery or at the time of surgery should be at minimal risk for osteoradionecrosis provided the tissues are handled carefully. When radiation therapy is planned as the sole treatment modality, there is a more urgent need to initiate therapy because delay allows tumor progression. A careful examination of the evidence proposed by Marx and Johnson delineated a dramatically decreased risk after 2 weeks. In this clinical setting, the author of this chapter found a 2-week period of healing to be adequate.

The treatment of patients after the development of osteoradionecrosis was standardized by an excellent report published by Marx.[12] In this report, he described the results obtained in 58 patients with the use of a standardized protocol for the management of osteoradionecrosis. Hyperbaric oxygen administration was combined with surgical therapy in a manner consistent with the clinical course of the disease process. Three stages of osteoradionecrosis therapy were described. Stage I involved the delivery of 30 hyperbaric oxygen therapy treatments followed by reevaluation. Success was defined as resorption of devitalized bone, granulation of the wound, and the absence of inflammation. Patients with improvement went on to a total of 60 dives. Persistent bone exposure, lack of mucosal healing, and persistent inflammation resulted in progression to stage II therapy.

Stage II therapy consisted of transoral alveolar sequestrectomy and primary mucosal closure with continued hyperbaric oxygen to 60 dives until clinical improvement was seen.

Wound dehiscence and bone exposure resulted in progression to stage III therapy. Likewise, patients with full-thickness (to the inferior border) bone resorption, pathologic fracture, or orocutaneous fistula proceeded to stage III.

Stage III therapy involved mandibular resection to bleeding bone and mandibular stabilization with primary closure. Hyperbaric oxygen was continued until a healthy mucosal closure was identified or to a total of 60 dives. Ten weeks after resection, patients were entered into stage III-R. Soft tissue deficits were corrected with pedicled muscle or myocutaneous flaps after 20 additional dives. Bone graft reconstruction was carried out in a transcutaneous approach followed by 10 additional hyperbaric oxygen treatments.

Marx used well-defined criteria for success in this treatment protocol. Of the 58 patients treated in this manner, nine were cured in stage I therapy, eight were cured in stage II, and 41 required stage III therapy. All reconstructions were ultimately successful. Total hyperbaric oxygen exposure time averaged 90 hours for stages I and II and 108 hours for stage III.

Summary

Radiation therapy will continue to play a significant role in the treatment of head and neck cancer. Dentists and surgeons can be useful in the care of patients with this type of cancer to prevent and manage complications. Through appropriate evaluation and timing of dental therapies prior to radiation therapy, osteoradionecrosis can be avoided. Additionally, application of good surgical principles to the management of the mandible during access osteotomies can limit the frequency and magnitude of postoperative healing difficulties.

The application of adjunctive measures to the dental and surgical treatment of patients following radiation therapy should be mandatory. Hyperbaric oxygen therapy has a well-defined role in the care of such patients. Failure to consider the positive effects of hyperbaric oxygen therapy prior to elective surgery in such patients constitutes practice outside of the standard of care. In the case of secondary mandibular reconstruction, the consideration of free tissue transfer to achieve mandibular continuity is recommended. If such expertise is not available, consideration for enhancement of free bone grafts with platelet-derived growth factors, in addition to standard protocol hyperbaric oxygen therapy, should be given.

The treatment of patients with head and neck cancer is indeed challenging. Particular attention to the application of evidence-based methods of practice will decrease the rate and magnitude of complications. However, complications are to be anticipated in these patients. Proper preparation, planning, and coordination of care delivery will limit the occurrence of complications and allow the surgeon and the patient to deal effectively with them and achieve satisfactory results.

References

1. Marx RE, Johnson RP. Studies in the radiobiology of osteoradionecrosis and their clinical significance. Oral Surg Oral Med Oral Pathol 1987;64:379.

2. Shah JP, Kumaraswamy SV, Kulkarni V. Comparative evaluation of fixation methods after mandibulotomy for oropharyngeal tumors. Am J Surg 1993;116:431.

3. Sullivan PK, Fabian R, Driscoll D. Mandibular osteotomies for tumor extirpation: The advantages of rigid fixation. Laryngoscope 1992;102:73.

4. Hunt TK, Dai MP. The effect of varying ambient oxygen tension on wound metabolism and collagen synthesis. Surg Gynecol Obstet 1972;135:561.

5. Knighton DR, Silver IA, Hunt TK. Regulation of wound angiogenesis: Effects of oxygen gradients and inspired oxygen concentrations. Surgery 1981;90:262.

6. Knighton DR, Hunt TK, Schenestuhl H. Oxygen tension regulates the expression of angiogenesis factor by macrophages. Science 1983;221:1283.

7. Marx RE, Ehler WJ, Tayapongsak P, Pierce LW. Relationship of oxygen dose to angiogenesis induction in irradiated tissue. Am J Surg 1990;160:519.

8. Marx RE, Johnson RP, Kline SN. Prevention of osteoradionecrosis: A randomized prospective clinical trial of hyperbaric oxygen versus penicillin. J Am Dent Assoc 1985;3:49.

9. Marx RE, Carlson ER, Eichstaedt RM, et al. Platelet-rich plasma growth factor enhancement for bone grafts. Oral Surg Oral Med Oral Pathol 1998;85:638.

10. Meyer I. Infectious diseases of the jaws. J Oral Surg 1970;28:17.

11. Marx RE. Osteoradionecrosis: A new concept of its pathophysiology. J Oral Maxillofac Surg 1983;41:283.

12. Marx RE. A new concept in the treatment of osteoradionecrosis. J Oral Maxillofac Surg 1983;41:351.

CHAPTER 14

Prosthodontic Reconstruction of the Hard and Soft Palate

Carl F. Driscoll, DMD

The reconstruction or rehabilitation of the patient undergoing a maxillectomy should start at diagnosis of the cancerous lesion. Most often, the initial health care provider who may have noticed a nonhealing lump, bump, or bleeding lesion is the general dentist. At this time, the patient is usually referred to an oral and maxillofacial surgeon or physician for evaluation and treatment. In addition to this referral, the general dentist should perform a thorough examination, including full-mouth radiographs and periodontal and endodontic evaluations. In the case of patients who undergo ablative surgery, the maintenance of teeth becomes paramount. The general dentist also should ensure that proper oral hygiene measures are maintained and that impressions are obtained for dental casts. These casts will be instrumental in the fabrication of fluoride trays, as well as in the planning of a surgical obturator for the patient.

Treatment of the cancerous lesion may include surgery, radiation, and chemotherapy, either alone or in combination. As the patient becomes more aware of the cancerous lesion, he or she realizes the severity of the situation.

The patient is confronted with the reality of being sick and must face that the illness may be terminal, or that the deformity or defect resulting from the treatment may leave hideous or grotesque results. All these factors can have a great impact on the psyche of the patient. The patient will need support from family, friends, and health care providers during this process. Professionalism, not pity, is required, especially from the physicians.

Treatments proposed and rendered should not be worse than the ailment, and the cure should not be worse than the illness. Hence, the quality of life issue is critical to the proposed treatment. Relatively speaking, the patient who has undergone a partial maxillectomy can be restored to normal appearance and function with a prosthesis following surgery. In many cases, prosthetic treatment is more desirable than surgical reconstruction in the patient who has had a maxillectomy.

The patient with a total maxillectomy (Fig 14-1) is the most difficult to treat prosthetically as well as emotionally. Function is always affected, and fabrication of the prosthesis is usually less than satisfactory to both the

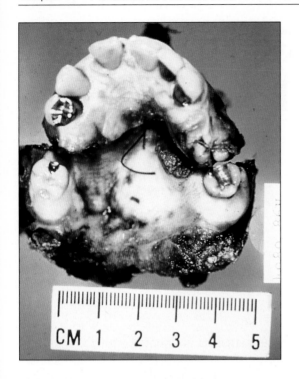

Fig 14-1 Removal of the entire maxilla.

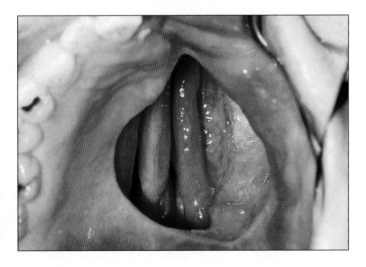

Fig 14-2 Example of a partial maxillectomy.

patient and the prosthodontist. The patient with a partial maxillectomy (Fig 14-2) is much easier to treat, depending on the remaining teeth and bony surfaces that can be saved. At diagnosis, all efforts should be made to save teeth for future retention, support, and stability of the prosthesis. This is far easier to accomplish before surgery rather than after.

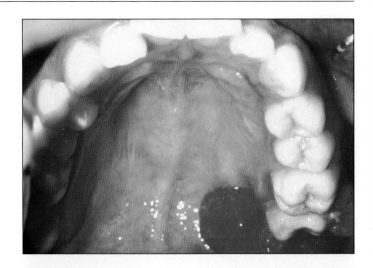

Fig 14-3 Maxillary ameloblastoma.

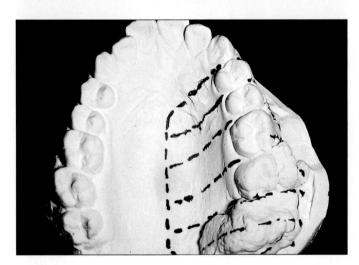

Fig 14-4 Dental cast with outline of proposed surgery.

Reconstructive Prostheses

Immediate obturator

An obturator is used to seal the remaining defect and restore function. As first described by Ambrose Pare, it is used to close a congenital or acquired tissue opening, primarily of the hard palate and/or contiguous alveolar structures.[1] It should be comfortable and restore adequate speech, mastication, and deglutition.[2] The obturator is normally fabricated by a maxillofacial prosthodontist or by a prosthodontist with additional training in this area.

Following the clinical (Fig 14-3) and radiographic examination of the patient, the surgeon meets with the prosthodontist to discuss the extent of the surgery. On study casts obtained earlier, the surgeon diagrams the proposed surgical site (Fig 14-4). With this

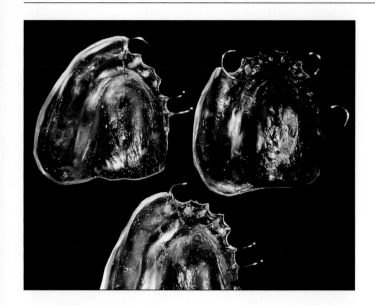

Fig 14-5 Multiple immediate obturators.

information, the prosthodontist fabricates an immediate obturator. This prosthesis is placed at surgery and serves the following functions: (1) acts as a matrix to hold the surgical packing in place; (2) reduces contamination of the surgical site; (3) enables the patient to speak more effectively by reproducing normal palatal contours; and (4) eases the psychological stress of the patient. All of these functions result in a much shorter hospital stay for the patient and hasten the recovery period.[3]

The patient awakening from anesthesia will not feel the defect, will be able to speak effectively, and will be able to take oral medications and food much earlier than if no immediate obturator is placed. This improves the patient's state of mind.

To improve the prosthetic prognosis, the surgeon places a split-thickness skin graft along the incision line in the mucobuccal fold. This graft limits the contracture of the scar band and increases the flexibility of the cheek.[2] Both results increase the success of the obturator dramatically. Often, the coronoid process is removed because it may interfere with the distobuccal extension of the obturator. Other fac-

tors that increase the success of the obturator are the retention of teeth, removal of nonfunctional soft palatal tissue, use of implants, and maintenance of as much of the hard palate as possible without sacrificing the integrity of the tumor margins during excision.

The obturator is designed without teeth and is held in place with clasps and/or wired in place. The flange of the obturator is designed to be short of the proposed skin graft–mucosa junction. The obturator is simple and lightweight and should follow normal palatal contours. Often, multiple immediate obturators are fabricated using different abutment teeth if the surgeon is not absolutely sure as to the anterior extent of the surgery (Fig 14-5). The obturator is left in place for 7 to 10 days, after which time the surgeon removes it and cleanses the surgical site. At this point, the patient usually realizes the severity of the surgery and the extent of the surgical defect, and then quickly realizes that speech is greatly affected and that food and fluid intake is impossible at this point. The use of clasps in the immediate obturator allows for a rapid conversion to an interim obturator.

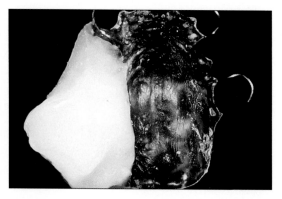

Fig 14-6 Immediate obturator relined with soft tissue liner to become an interim obturator.

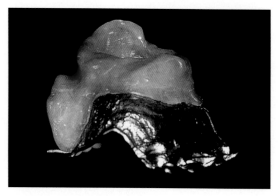

Fig 14-7 Definitive obturator.

Interim obturator

After the immediate obturator is removed, it is relined with soft tissue reline material to aid in retention of the prosthesis (Fig 14-6). The interim obturator is removed by the patient daily for cleansing and tissue recovery. As with all soft tissue liners, home care is crucial to maintaining the longevity of the liner. Teeth may be added to the interim obturator at a later appointment for psychological, more than functional, reasons.

If no immediate obturator is available, a delayed obturator may be fabricated. This is made 7 to 10 days after surgery. An existing prosthesis may be used in this method. Disadvantages of the delayed obturator include discomfort to the patient during the manipulation of tissues at this stage of healing and loss of the advantages that were listed previously for an immediate obturator.

Definitive obturator

Following tissue healing—usually 6 months or more—fabrication of a more definitive obturator commences. The definitive obturator resembles a removable partial denture with a bulb on

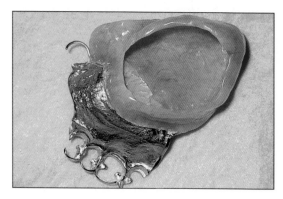

Fig 14-8 Hollowed bulb on a definitive obturator.

top (Fig 14-7). The framework is fabricated in a manner similar to that of a conventional removable partial denture with the defect being recorded with modeling plastic and a wash of a light body impression material, a mouth temperature wax, or tissue conditioner. Often the bulb portion of the obturator is hollowed out to decrease the weight of the prosthesis (Fig 14-8). Wu and Schaaf[4] reported that up to a 33% reduction of weight may be attained with this procedure. Maintenance of the definitive obturator is the same as that for a removable partial denture with regard to removal for 8 hours a day and cleansing techniques.

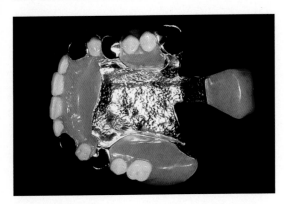

Fig 14-9 Obturator with soft palate extension (cameo view).

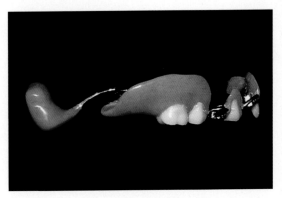

Fig 14-10 Obturator with soft palate extension (lateral view).

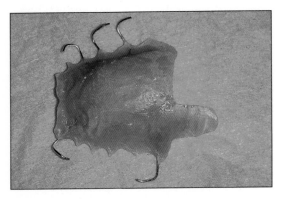

Fig 14-11 Palatal lift prosthesis on cast.

Obturator with soft palate extension

Patients with lesions involving the soft palate that require excision need a different mode of treatment[5] (Fig 14-9). With speech dependent on the movement of not only the soft palate but also the lateral and posterior pharyngeal walls, the fabrication of a prosthesis is much more difficult. The prosthesis must be fabricated to allow for air passage around the pha-

ryngeal extension of the obturator during certain speech sounds (Fig 14-10). The impression of this area must be obtained under function using the materials listed previously. A functional seal is also desirable. Patients who have no lateral or posterior pharyngeal wall movement will have a less than ideal result. Obviously, with an extension, which is required to replace the soft palate, the retention of teeth is critical. Edentulous patients may require adhesives to maintain the prosthesis, depending on the size of the pharyngeal extension.

Palatal lift prosthesis

Patients who have an intact but nonfunctional soft palate may be candidates for a palatal lift prosthesis[6] (Fig 14-11). This prosthesis is useful in patients who have diminished or absent motor function due to cerebrovascular trauma, myasthenia gravis, bulbar poliomyelitis, or cerebral palsy.[3] The function of the palatal prosthesis is to mechanically lift the soft palate to its normal position during function to allow for the constricture of the lateral and posterior pharyngeal walls to accomplish closure (Fig 14-12). Contraindications to the use of the

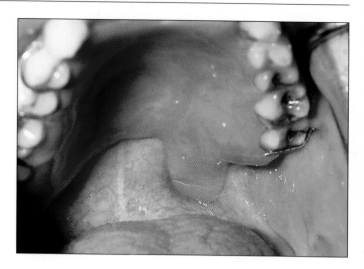

Fig 14-12 Palatal lift prosthesis intra-orally.

palatal lift prosthesis include a noncompliant patient, nonfunctional pharyngeal walls, lack of retention, and a palate that cannot be displaced superiorly.

Summary

The techniques described in this chapter require the expertise of an experienced prosthodontist; however, the general dentist is important in the initial detection of the cancerous lesion, initial handling of the patient in terms of caries control, and long-term routine oral care.

Patients will continue to live long prosperous lives after the cancer treatment has been completed, and their dental care must not be neglected. It is imperative that the general dentist become more aware of the treatment needs of these patients to help the prosthodontist fabricate the previously mentioned prostheses and to improve patients' quality of life.

References

1. Glossary of Prosthodontic Terms, ed 6. J Prosthet Dent 1994;71:87.
2. Desjardins R. Obturator prosthesis design for acquired maxillary defects. J Prosthet Dent 1978;39:424–435.
3. Beumer J, Curtis T, Marunick M. Maxillofacial Rehabilitation: Prosthodontic and Surgical Considerations. St Louis: Ishiyaku EuroAmerica, 1996:240.
4. Wu Y, Schaaf N. Comparison of weight reduction in different designs of solid and hollow obturator prostheses. J Prosthet Dent 1989;62:214–217.
5. Beder O. Fundamentals for maxillofacial prosthetics. Springfield, IL: Thomas, 1974:171.
6. Gibbons P, Bloomer H. A supportive-type prosthetic speech aid. J Prosthet Dent 1958;8:362–369.

CHAPTER 15

The Role of Implant-Supported Prostheses

Marvin L. Baer, DDS, MS, and Remy H. Blanchaert, Jr, MD, DDS

Surgical treatment modalities are commonly used in the treatment of patients with cancers of the oral cavity. The extent of the surgery required for the extirpation of disease can vary from small soft tissue defects to large composite (bone and soft tissue) defects. These resections present many challenges to those charged with restoration of normal function and cosmesis. Reconstructive surgery and osseointegrated implants are combined in this endeavor. Oral rehabilitation significantly improves the quality of life for these patients. The challenges and complexity encountered in the rehabilitation of patients following surgical therapy for oral cancer are myriad. This chapter is intended to arm the dentist with the necessary knowledge and skills to contribute to the well-being of the patient with oral cancer.

Treatment Considerations

In the treatment of patients with cancers of the oral cavity, the restorative dentist is confront-ed with unique challenges. Major advances in surgical technique have resulted in better restoration of orofacial form through the increased use of free tissue transfer. Despite the best efforts of the reconstructive surgeon, the restorative dentist will continue to identify significant deviations from normal anatomy in both bone and soft tissue. No reconstruction can restore the tissues to the exact pre-morbid condition. Typically the restorative dentist encounters deficiencies in supporting bone in the neomandible, thick mobile tissue overlying the neomandible, and decreased or absent vestibular depth with minimal distensibility. Muscle attachments have often been modified and result in abrupt limits to the oral prosthesis. The surgical reconstruction often results in less than ideal ridge relationships and interarch distance.

Additional adjunct therapies, such as chemotherapy and radiation therapy, also affect the health of the lining tissues of the oral cavity. These alterations (xerostomia, mucosal atrophy, fungal infection, ulceration, and an abnormal wound-healing response) further complicate oral restoration.

Advantages of implants

Because of these abnormalities, osseointegrated implants are extremely useful to the dentist and offer several advantages for postsurgical oral tumor patients. These advantages are:

1. Rigid stabilization of the dental appliance to the supporting bone
2. Support for the prosthesis, reducing unwanted pressure on compromised and soft tissues
3. Decreased reliance on the patient's oral coordination, which is often impaired

Osseointegrated implant placement in patients with oral cancer is complicated by the alteration in the tissues from normal as previously listed. Especially important in this regard is the effect of radiation therapy on the wound healing response and therefore implant integration. The results of studies identify several important factors in the successful integration of osseointegrated implants in irradiated bone. As early as 1993 reports began to appear linking radiation to decreased implant integration. Granstrom et al[1] reported increased loss of implants placed in irradiated native bone but demonstrated long-term success in those implants that survived the first few years following placement. Their group has been responsible for several excellent works studying the effects of radiation and hyperbaric oxygen therapy on the integration of dental and craniofacial implants in patients with irradiated cancer. They have demonstrated improvement in implant survival rates in patients who receive hyperbaric oxygen therapy and a correlation between increasing radiation dose and increasing rates of implant failure.[2] Many other authors also have written on this topic.[3-6] A summary of the data supports the placement of implants in patients who receive radiation therapy for oral cancer when

clinically indicated. Overengineering of the reconstruction (ie, increased number of implants placed) and the selective use of hyperbaric oxygen therapy are prudent modifications from standard treatment regimens.

Dental rehabilitation of patients with head and neck cancer using osseointegrated implants in sites of mandibular reconstruction has been reported as well. Foster et al[7] reported an 83% success rate for implants placed in nonvascularized bone graft reconstructions. Urken et al[8] reported an 86% success rate for osseointegrated implants placed at the time of primary microvascular mandibular reconstruction (simultaneous with ablative surgery) with subsequent irradiation.

As previously stated, the postsurgical patient may present with problems in ridge relationship or constricted soft tissue. Bone grafting may provide needed support but sometimes results in diminished interarch space. The location of implants may be complicated as a result of these and other reconstructive problems. Compromised implant location and angulation requires unique, inventive solutions.

A wide variety of prosthetic components have been developed to deal with misalignment of implant fixtures. Custom abutments also help solve some of the unusual problems presented by patients previously deemed untreatable prior to the development of osseointegrated implants.

Diagnosis and treatment planning

Careful diagnosis and treatment planning are very important to achieve a predictable result. The team approach among the restorative dentist, the surgeon, the laboratory, and the patient add immeasurably to achieving success in implant rehabilitation for all patients, but especially for the complexities encountered in the cancer patient. Diagnostic imaging to include panoramic radiography and/or computed tomography (CT) scans are of paramount importance to allow understanding of changes in hard tissue wrought by the surgical intervention in these patients. Only CT scans provide three-dimensional insight into problems that may occur if only conventional two-dimensional radiographs are available.

An integral part of communication among the team members is the diagnostic waxup or setup and the surgical guide. The diagnostic waxup provides the opportunity to analyze the biomechanics of the reconstruction including the occlusion, orientation of the occlusal plane, and tooth length and position. This area of diagnosis is the basis for communication between the restorative dentist and the laboratory technician. Only after a careful analysis of the diagnostic waxup can decisions be made about implant number, location, and angulation. At this point careful discussion between the restorative dentist and the surgeon is necessary to discover the feasibility of ideal implant placement relative to the bony framework.

Compromises are often needed to achieve a workable treatment plan for the patient. After decisions are made about implant placement, the surgical guide is constructed to communicate this information in a workable form to the surgeon at the time of implant surgery. Even with the most carefully made surgical guide available, it is strongly advisable for the restorative dentist to be present at the time of implant placement surgery. Unforeseen problems almost always arise requiring on-the-spot decisions during surgery. In spite of careful planning, the restorative dentist's viewpoint needs to be provided. An improperly placed implant is often worse than no implant when rehabilitation procedures begin. The value of the team approach to treatment of these complex cases cannot be overemphasized. The additional time required pays dividends when the final results are realized.

Prosthesis design

Two primary types of prosthesis are generally considered for the postsurgical patient: the hybrid prosthesis and the overdenture. The hybrid prosthesis is similar to the type designed by Dr Brånemark as part of his original research and provides the greatest functional improvement for patients (Box 15-1). This appliance is screwed into place and removable only by the dentist. Its design allows for brushing, flossing, and other hygiene measures (Fig 15-1). Soft tissue trauma after radiation therapy can be a major problem but is also decreased with this implant-supported design.[9]

Box 15-1 Hybrid Prostheses	
Advantages	**Disadvantages**
Permanently fixed	Patient maintenance is more difficult
No pressure on soft tissue	Not as easily modified
Borders are short of muscle attachments	No flange for lip support
Patient feels more "whole"	Cannot be removed for cleaning

The overdenture approach (Box 15-2) provides a more flexible approach to reconstructive treatment (Fig 15-2a). This appliance may be supported by a gold bar with Hader clips or other types of attachments (Fig 15-2b). Individual attachments such as the ERA or ball attachment are used in other circumstances (Figs 15-3a and 15-3b). When the overdenture design uses two implants with or without a connecting bar, support is provided by both implants and soft tissue. When four or more implants are used to support a longer connecting bar, the overdenture can be designed to be exclusively implant supported (Figs 15-4a and 15-4b).

Box 15-2 Overdentures

Advantages	Disadvantages
Especially indicated for obturator appliances	Need more prosthetic space for components
Allows flange for lip support	Not as secure during function
More easily modified	Patient more aware of defect
Removable for cleaning	
More latitude for implant misalignment	

Because of the possibility of cancer recurrence, especially during the first 3 years after tumor removal, treatment planning should include provisions for change and modification. Placement of additional implant fixtures to help provide maximum flexibility is an excellent principle for treatment in the oral cancer patient.

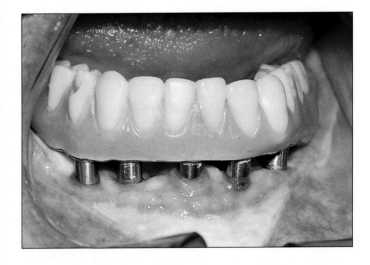

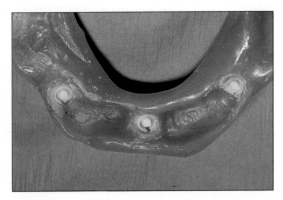

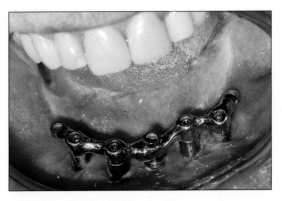

Fig 15-1 The hybrid prosthesis, a screw-retained prosthesis often used to restore the edentulous mandible.

Fig 15-2a The internal surface of an implant-supported overdenture with three ERA male attachments.

Fig 15-2b The implant-supported connecting bar with three ERA female attachments that support the overdenture shown in Fig 15-2a.

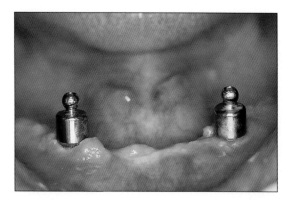

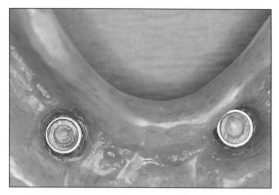

Fig 15-3a Individual ball attachments that screw directly into the implant fixtures.

Fig 15-3b Internal surface of an implant-supported overdenture, which is supported by ball attachments as shown in Fig 15-3a.

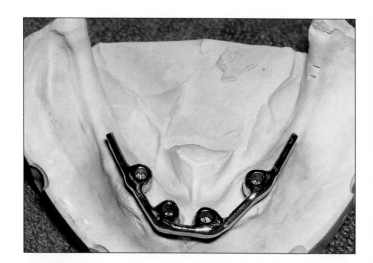

Fig 15-4a Implant connecting bar supported by four implants with sufficient anteroposterior spread to make the denture totally implant supported.

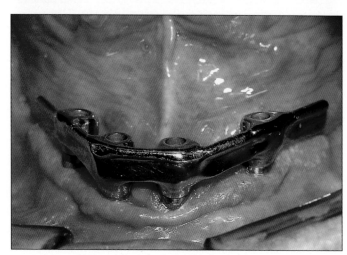

Fig 15-4b Implant connecting bar in the mouth. Four Hader clips provide retention for the denture.

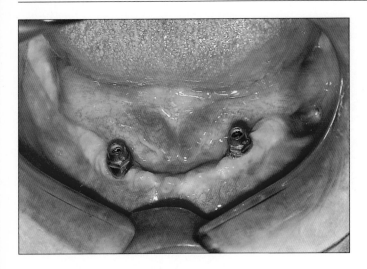

Fig 15-5a Two ERA direct overdenture abutments, which can be obtained to fit most implant fixtures.

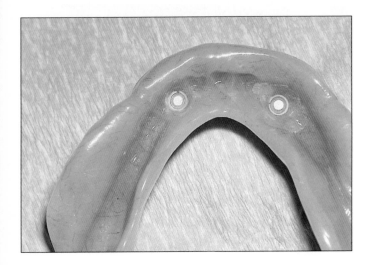

Fig 15-5b The implant overdenture with two ERA male attachments, which is placed with two implants, as shown in Fig 15-5a.

Clinical Examples

Examples of patient treatment range from simple to complex. A small simple-looking reconstruction can master many challenges (Fig 15-5a). For example, a completely edentulous patient underwent removal of a tumor in the area of the left mandibular molars 20 years ago. The defect was small but significant because the patient was edentulous. Any mandibular complete denture results in a major loss in function. The additional defect from the excision of the ameloblastoma caused additional problems for the patient. With two implant fixtures in the right and left canine areas, ERA attachments were placed in the implant fixtures with no connecting bar. Two plastic male attachments placed in the mandibular complete overdenture (Fig 15-5b) resulted in a significant improvement in function.

Surgery for the removal of a verrucous carcinoma required a rim resection of the mandibu-

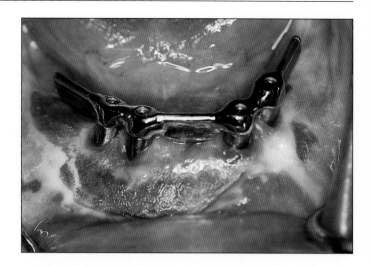

Fig 15-6a An implant connecting bar, with two segments cantilevered distal to the most distal implants.

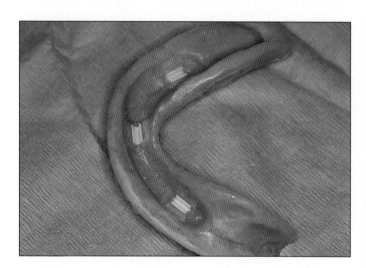

Fig 15-6b Internal surface of the overdenture with three Hader clips that attach to the connecting bar shown in Fig 15-6a.

lar alveolar ridge. A skin graft and vestibuloplasty were later performed to gain attached tissue for the remaining residual ridge. Although the surgical result was excellent, the resulting defect would have been difficult to manage with a conventional complete denture. Four implant fixtures were placed with emphasis on a good anteroposterior spread. Wide distribution of the implants allowed for a screw-retained bar with the distal portion of the bar cantilevered behind the most distal implants

(Fig 15-6a). An overdenture with three Hader clips provided excellent retention and support for the prosthesis (Fig 15-6b).

In another patient, three separate lesions of squamous cell carcinoma occurred over a 10-year period, with two lesions in the mandible resulting in a resection of the body of the mandible from the area of the right first premolar to the left ramus. The woman was 85 years old at the time of the resection. All remaining mandibular teeth were lost at that

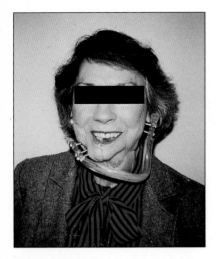

Fig 15-7a Patient with external fixation (Joe Hall Morris splint) following resection of more than half of the body of the mandible.

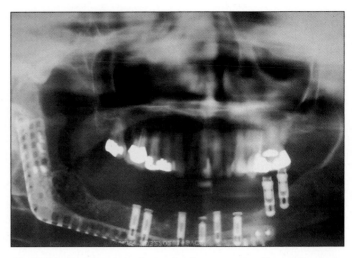

Fig 15-7b Panoramic radiograph after reconstruction of the body of the mandible followed by placement of six implants in the site. Two implants on the left side had been placed previously.

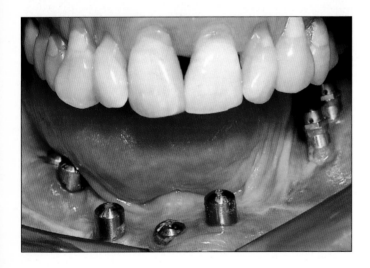

Fig 15-7c Clinical view of implants after placement of healing abutments. All implants were not used in the original reconstruction that followed.

time. A Joe Hall Morris splint (Fig 15-7a) was placed to fix the remaining left condyle and remaining right segment of the mandible. About 2 months later, a Timesh titanium basket and autogenous bone graft from the iliac crest were placed to reconstruct the mandible.

About 6 months later, six osseointegrated implants were placed in the grafted site (Fig 15-7b). The surgeon placed more implants than required, because the age and health of the patient meant that further implant surgery might not be possible (Fig 15-7c). The concept

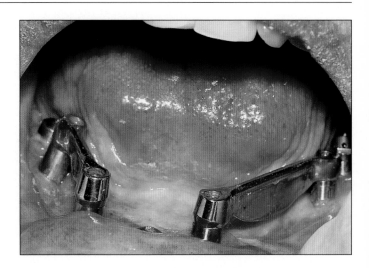

Fig 15-7d Placement of two gold bars supported by four implants.

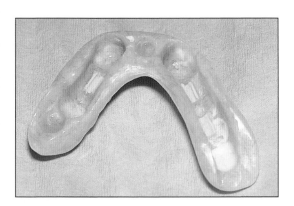

Fig 15-7e Implant-supported prosthesis showing three Hader clips that attach to the bar.

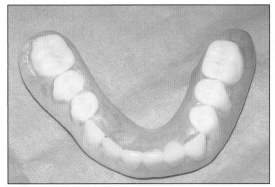

Fig 15-7f Occlusal view of the implant prosthesis.

of overengineering is important in patients with cancer, especially in patients who are older and in fragile health. Prosthetic reconstruction consisted of two gold bars supported by four implant fixtures (Fig 15-7d). An overdenture was constructed and retained by three Hader clips (Figs 15-7e and 15-7f). Loss of some implants as a result of an infection 2 years later resulted in loss of the gold bars. However, the prosthesis support was maintained by placement of individual ERA attachments on remaining implant fixtures.

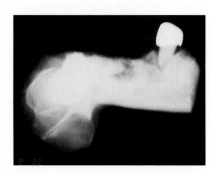

Fig 15-8a A radiograph of a segment of the mandible removed to resect a large ameloblastoma.

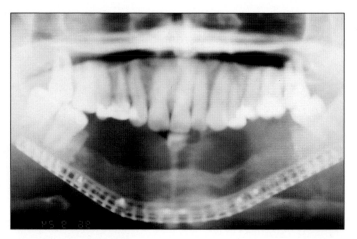

Fig 15-8b Reconstruction of the mandible immediately following resection. A Timesh titanium basket filled with particulate bone marrow harvested from the ilium is used to restore the defect.

Clinical Procedure

Resection of a large mandibular tumor that had been treated by conservative means for many years resulted in removal of the mandible anterior to the right and left second molars (Fig 15-8a). The mandible was reconstructed at the time of resection with a Timesh titanium basket and a particulate marrow graft from the patient's posterior ilium (Fig 15-8b). A hybrid prosthesis was selected as the treatment of choice to provide the best functional result. Six months later, the prosthodontist made jaw relation records, mounted casts, determined the best positioning of the replacement teeth, and constructed a surgical guide (Fig 15-8c) to aid in the placement of six osseointegrated implant fix-

tures in the grafted area (Figs 15-8d and 15-8e). The patient had natural teeth in the maxilla opposing the prosthesis, which made the location of implant fixtures more critical. The implants were widely spaced since there was no concern for the nonexistent inferior alveolar canal. After 6 months of healing, the implant fixtures were uncovered and prosthodontic treatment was initiated. Impressions were taken and a verification jig was made to confirm the accuracy of the impression (Fig 15-8f). The frame was tried in and the fit verified (Fig 15-8g). The final prosthesis was placed (Fig 15-8h). The patient had lost his mandibular teeth more than 20 years ago and was very happy with the improved function of a fixed, screw-retained prosthesis (Fig 15-8i).

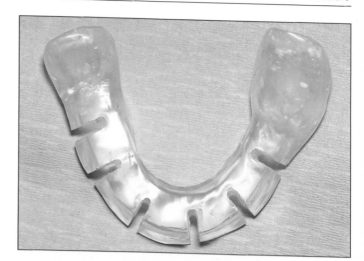

Fig 15-8c A surgical guide made by the prosthodontist, in consultation with the surgeon, to aid in the location of the implant fixtures about 6 months after mandibular reconstruction.

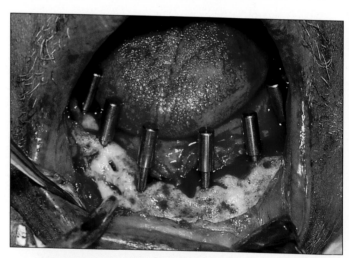

Fig 15-8d Implant guide pins in place after all implant holes have been drilled. Alignment is directed slightly lingual because of the relatively larger size of the mandible in comparison to the maxilla.

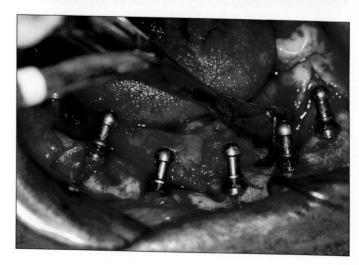

Fig 15-8e Implants at the time of placement. Placement tools are still in position.

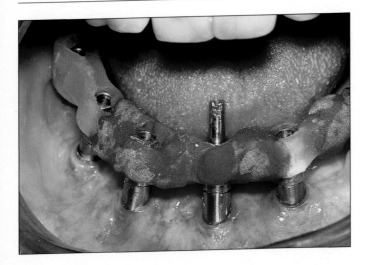

Fig 15-8f Prosthodontic phase. A verification jig in position to verify the accuracy of the cast.

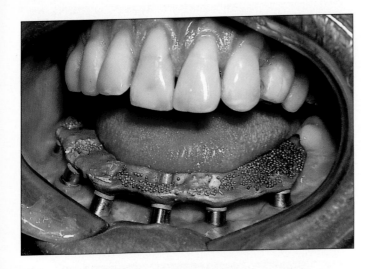

Fig 15-8g Frame try-in to verify the accuracy of the frame to the implants.

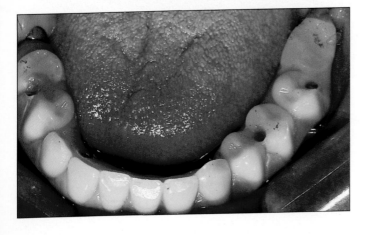

Fig 15-8h Final prosthesis at the time of delivery. The occlusal rest of the natural molar was later removed to avoid the possibility of caries in that area.

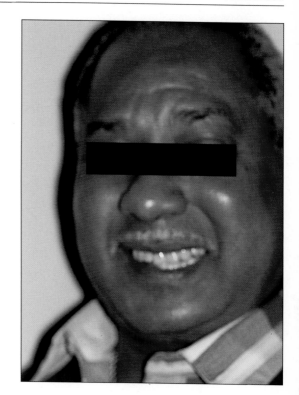

Fig 15-8i Facial view of patient after placement of the final restoration.

References

1. Granstrom G, Tjellström A, Brånemark P-I, Fornamder J. Bone-anchored reconstruction of the irradiated head and neck cancer patient. Otolaryngol Head Neck Surg 1993;108:334.

2. Granstrom G. The use of hyperbaric oxygen to prevent implant loss in the irradiated patient. In: Worthington R, Brånemark P-I (eds). Advanced Osseointegrated Surgery: Applications in the Maxillofacial Region. Chicago: Quintessence, 1992:336–345.

3. Taylor TD, Worthington P. Osseointegrated implant rehabilitation of the previously irradiated mandible: Results of a limited trial at 3 to 7 years. J Prosthet Dent 1993;69:60.

4. Franzen L, Rosenquist JB, Rosenquist KI, Gustafsson I. Oral implant rehabilitation of patients with oral malignancies treated with radiation therapy and surgery without adjunctive hyperbaric oxygen. Int J Oral Maxillofac Implants 1995;10:183.

5. Niimi A, Fujimoto T, Nosaka Y, Ueda M. A Japanese multicenter study of osseointegrated implants placed in irradiated tissues: A preliminary report. Int J Oral Maxillofac Implants 1997;12:259.

6. Anderson G, Andreasson L, Bjelkengren G. Oral implant rehabilitation in irradiated patients without adjunctive hyperbaric oxygen. Int J Oral Maxillofac Implants 1998;13:647.

7. Foster RD, Anthony JP, Sharma A, Pogrel MA. Vascularized bone flaps versus nonvascularized bone grafts for mandibular reconstruction: An outcome analysis of primary bony union and endosseous implant success. Head Neck 1999;21:66.

8. Urken ML, Buchbinder D, Costantino PD, et al. Oromandibular reconstruction using microvascular composite flaps. Arch Otolaryngol Head Neck Surg 1998;124:46.

9. Weischer T, Schettler D, Mohr C. Concepts of surgical and implant supported prosthesis in the rehabilitation of patients with oral cancer. Int J Oral Maxillofac Implants 1996;11:775.

CHAPTER 16

Speech Production and Swallowing

M. Cara Erskine, MEd

Speech production and swallowing function are interconnected processes. The same structures play a part in each complex act.

Speech Production

Speech production is divided into three main parts: respiration, phonation, and articulation. These processes function together in synchrony for speech production. Respiration is responsible for vibration of the vocal folds, which in turn provides the sound source. The resonated sound is refined by the vocal tract, which consists of the area from the vocal folds to the lips and is actually a series of chambers. The vocal tract is a complex system that makes adjustments for the different sounds of speech. The change that occurs in the production of each sound is attributed to the dynamic movement of the structures during speech production (Fig 16-1). Although not indispensable, the tongue is generally thought to be the most influential structure for speech production. Other main structures include the mandible, hard and soft palate, teeth, and lips.

Intelligibility depends on the changes of the vocal tract and the regularity of the movement. There are 25 consonants and 14 vowels and diphthongs that are basic elements of speech. Speech production is divided into where the constriction takes place and the manner of articulation, which is the type of acoustic event as the articulators are moved.

Swallowing

Swallowing is a complex chain of events that occurs to transport food safely from the mouth into the esophagus. It is broken down into four phases: oral preparatory—the food is manipulated in the mouth; oral—the tongue pushes the food posteriorly; pharyngeal—the swallow reflex is initiated and the bolus is moved through the pharynx; and esophageal—the food is moved through the esophagus once it passes through the cricopharyngeal segment (Fig 16-2). The first three stages can be affected by oral cancer treatment and are usually manageable by therapeutic techniques as directed by a speech language pathologist. Logemann[2]

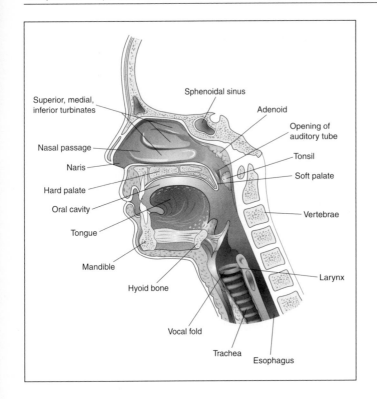

Fig 16-1 The vocal tract. (From Palmer and Yantis[1].)

reports that, with a change in head and body posture, swallowing is improved in 75% to 80% of patients with dysphagia.

Oral cancer accounts for approximately 8% of all malignant disease.[3] The tongue accounts for 26% of all oral cancers and 0.7% of all cancers.[4] Most often, it is seen in the fifth and sixth decades of life. It is also considered one of the most devastating cancers, because it causes impairments in communication and swallowing skills, thus contributing to significant psychosocial issues. Tumors occurring in the oral cavity are managed with surgery and/or radiation therapy and may or may not require chemotherapy. The type and degree of treatment affect the outcome of speech and swallowing due to the involvement of the oral cavity structures. The changes that are encountered usually require assessment and treatment by a speech language pathologist as part of the multidisciplinary team workup.

This enables the patient to return to as normal a functional level as possible. Generally, the more structures that are taken, the less mobile and sensate the remaining tissue and the greater the rehabilitation challenge for the speech language pathologist.

Role of the Speech Language Pathologist

The speech language pathologist is an integral part of the rehabilitation team, which consists of a social worker, nutritionist, dentist, prosthodontist, oral maxillofacial surgeon, oncologist, medical doctor, and nursing staff. Typically, the patient's case is discussed in the multidisciplinary meeting and treatment options are considered. The speech language pathologist provides integral information about

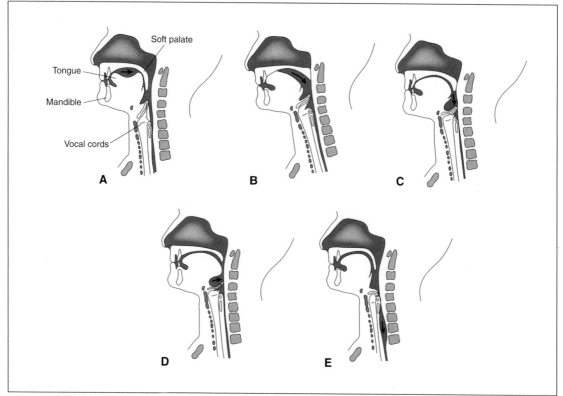

Fig 16-2 Lateral view of bolus propulsion during the swallow. (A) The voluntary initiation of the swallow by the tongue; (B) the triggering of the pharyngeal swallow; (C) the arrival of the bolus in the vallecula; (D) the tongue base retraction to the anteriorly moving pharyngeal wall; and (E) the bolus in the cervical esophagus and cricopharyngeal region. (From Logemann[2].)

the expected rehabilitation plan and possible outcome (Box 16-1). When the patient is seen for the preoperative assessment, a speech and swallowing screening is conducted; counseling regarding the types of problems that may be encountered is provided; and the treatment plan is discussed. If needed, a modified barium swallowing examination is arranged. Frequently, the full impact of the surgery is not known until it is completed. However, it is important that the patient and family are made aware that there are speech language pathologists with expertise in facilitating the critical aspects of the rehabilitation plan (Box 16-2).

The patient is informed that exercise is a critical part of the rehabilitation plan for which he or she is responsible.

Outcome studies are limited for patients with oral cancer, as such studies usually examine a small number of patients with multiple surgery sites and thus provide limited information on the reconstruction.[5] There is thus no precise information about the influence of treatment on speech and swallowing function. It can be predicted, however, that the greater the percentage of tongue and base of the tongue that is resected, the more significant the effect on swallowing and speech.[6]

Box 16-1 Speech Language Pathologist's Role in Rehabilitation

Preoperative
Input into the expected postoperative treatment plan
Baseline assessment of speech and swallowing
Advice to patient about the postoperative plan and the importance of practicing oral motor exercises

Postoperative
Baseline assessment to determine readiness for initiation of oral intake
Assessment of communication skills
Modified barium swallow exam
Provision of therapy for speech and swallowing daily for an inpatient and weekly for an outpatient

At Discharge
Establishment of a plan for follow-up on speech and swallowing skills for an outpatient
Cooperation with other disciplines

Box 16-2 Swallowing and Speech Therapy Strategies

Adaptive utensils for food presentation for improved positioning and allowing for modification of volumes presented
Postural changes for improvement in the flow of the bolus
Changes in food consistency (liquid, paste, solid)
Prosthesis
Exercises to improve airway protection and range of motion
Prosthesis and exercises will also be used for speech improvement.

Box 16-3   Surgery Type and Expected Impact on Swallowing and Speech

Removal of < 50% of the tongue	Temporary problems due to swelling and decreased sensation; full recovery expected; speech generally shows good intelligibility
Removal of > 50% of the tongue	Reduced oral control, which may lead to decreased oral transport; speech shows fair to good intelligibility
Composite resection	Reduced oral control, residual material in the oral cavity, delayed initiation of the swallow reflex, decreased pharyngeal wall movement; speech shows fair to moderately impaired intelligibility
Total glossectomy with flap	Inability to control anything in the oral cavity; absent sensation in the flap area; inability to generate adequate pressure to force material through the pharynx; reduced laryngeal excursion; speech shows severe to moderate impairment

Massengill et al[3] stated that the larger the amount of tongue removed, the poorer the speech. However, one patient had 95% of his tongue removed and "was still able to communicate fairly well."[3] Determining the outcome for the treatment given to an individual patient is not possible, however.

Once the patient has undergone surgery, the speech language pathologist usually sees him or her several days postoperatively to answer any questions. The speech language pathologist needs to know the type and degree of the resection and the reconstruction technique that was performed. When the surgery involves 50% or less of the tongue with no other structures and a primary closure is used, the difficulties are often temporary (Box 16-3). If the volume of tongue removed is greater than 50%, the effects are magnified.[1] Although the tongue volume and surrounding structures play a role in speech production and swallowing, it is not known what amount of tissue mass is required to achieve normality in these functions.[7] Remarkably, some patients gain reasonably intelligible speech, thus the tongue may not be indispensable. Tongue resection reduces bulk and mobility, resulting in impaired articulation and swallowing, especially in the oral stages. If the tongue tip is removed, speech is most affected.[8] Skelly et al[9] looked at intelligibility after speech therapy in patients who had undergone partial glossectomies and total glossectomies and had scores of 0% and 8%, respectively, before therapy. After speech therapy, the scores increased to 18% and 42%, respectively. Treatment focused on lengthening vowel duration, reducing intensity, integrating meaningful pauses, and elevating pitch.[9]

In swallowing, if 50% or more of the tongue is removed, patients will have diminished oral control. They generally do best with liquids and thin paste and usually rely on gravity to move the material through the oral cavity.

Therapy is focused on range-of-motion exercises for the tongue, and patients may benefit from a prosthesis to lower the palatal vault, which decreases the height, helping to move material through the oral cavity and contributing to better control.

Special Considerations

Anterior floor of the mouth resection

If the tongue is mobile, minimal problems are noted and they are usually temporary. If the tongue is sutured into the defect, creating severe mobility problems, speech and swallowing problems are significant. Liquid syringed to the posterior tongue may be the best method. The use of a flap for closure provides a more mobile tongue with better control, leading to an increased ability to manage the bolus. The tongue needs to be freely mobile to handle materials other than liquids. If there is a lateral floor of the mouth, base of the tongue, and posterior floor of the mouth resection, the oral and pharyngeal stage of swallowing may be involved. Patients may experience oral stage swallowing problems, difficulty triggering the swallow reflex, poor base of tongue retraction, and diminished pharyngeal wall movement. Dysphagia is the worst after surgery on the floor of the mouth, base of the tongue, and lateral pharyngeal wall.[10] A palatal prosthesis can contribute to an improvement in swallowing by lowering the palatal vault, which gives better control of the bolus and increases the speed of the swallow. The risk of aspiration is reduced and therefore allows for greater variability of tolerance. Speech also improves with a prosthesis which can aid in closing the velopharyngeal deficit and lowering the palatal configuration, allowing for better tongue contact. There may be changes over time requiring adjustments to the device.[11]

Radiation therapy

Radiation therapy presents another dilemma for swallowing. It contributes to reduced saliva, edema, and mucositis. These in turn contribute to oral stage swallowing problems. Fibrosis can continue for years. The pharyngeal stage can be affected if it is in the radiation field, and can cause problems with the triggering of the reflex. Generally, the higher the dosage, the poorer the swallowing function. The importance of continued oral motor exercises needs to be stressed to patients so mobility is maximized.

Treatment

Speech and swallowing therapy are tailored to each patient based on the specific identified problems following surgery. It is impossible to predict how patients will perform until they are given a postoperative speech and swallowing assessment. Usually, the initial assessment is performed on patients 3 to 14 days after surgery. The evaluation consists of clinical assessment of the oral structures, bedside assessment of swallowing, an articulation skills assessment, and a modified barium swallow examination with trial of treatment strategies. The main dysphagia symptoms following oral cancer resections include reduced oral control, inadequate lip function, poor chewing, poor velopharyngeal seal, reduced tongue strength/range of motion, delayed initiation of swallow reflex, reduced laryngeal excursion, and reduced pharyngeal movement. Any of these can lead to aspiration.

After the treatment strategies, which may include oral motor exercises and safe swallowing techniques such as positioning and/or airway protection guidelines, are outlined, the patient is seen daily in hospital for continued efforts to improve both speech and swallowing skills. Oral motor exercises are instituted to improve range of motion for the oral structures. A modified barium swallow examination is performed so that problems can be noted and compensatory strategies considered to determine what food consistencies are safe to resume.

If 50% or less of the tongue is removed, speech will be quite intelligible. If more than 50% is resected, it will be fair, and as more structures are involved, it will become poorer. If a total glossectomy is performed, an augmentative device, such as a Canon communicator, should be considered.

Prosthetics are another necessary aspect of the speech and swallowing rehabilitation process. They need to be introduced early to move the patient to rehabilitation more quickly. The prosthesis helps with improving the lingual palatal contact, thus allowing for improvement in speech production and oral control of the bolus.[12] Early use is thought to reduce the development of bad habits.

Speech and swallowing therapy is aimed at increasing the mobility of the affected structures and determining what compensatory strategies will aid in improving both aspects. Working closely with the prosthodontist helps to obtain the best fit to maximize function. Working with the patient through the radiation treatment to maintain function is always necessary.

Rehabilitation is an ongoing process and changes can be noted long after the initial therapy. Better tracking of the different types of treatment and the outcome is necessary so that there is a better knowledge base to effectively treat patients who undergo this devastating surgery. It is in the best interests of these patients that they are treated via a multidisciplinary team approach.

References

1. Palmer JM, Yantis PA. Survey of Communication Disorders. Baltimore, MD: Williams and Wilkins, 1990.

2. Logemann JA. Evaluation and Treatment of Swallowing Disorders, ed 2. Austin, TX: Pro-Ed, 1998.

3. Massengill R, Maxwell S, Pickrell K. An analysis of articulation following partial and total glossectomy. J Speech Hear Disord 1970;35:170–173.

4. Davis JW, Lazarus C, Logemann J, Hurst PS. Effect of maxillary glossectomy prosthesis on articulation and swallowing. J Prosthet Dent 1987;57:715–719.

5. Pauloski BR, Logemann JA, Rademaker AW, McConnel FM, Heiser MA, Cardinale S, et al. Speech and swallowing function after anterior tongue and floor of mouth resection with distal flap reconstruction. J Speech Hear Res 1993;36:267–276.

6. McConnel FMS, Logemann JA, Rademaker AW, et al. Surgical variables affecting postoperative swallowing efficiency in oral cancer patients: A pilot study. Laryngoscope 1994;104:87–90.

7. Urken ML, Moscoso JF, Lawson W, Biller HF. A systematic approach to functional reconstruction of the oral cavity following partial and total glossectomy. Arch Otolaryngol Head Neck Surg 1994;120: 589–601.

8. Robbins KT, Bowman JB, Jacob RF. Postglossectomy deglutitory and articulatory rehabilitation with palatal augmentation prosthesis. Arch Otolaryngol Head Neck Surg 1987;113:1214–1218.

9. Skelly M, Donaldson RC, Fust RS, Seelye BJ. Glossectomy Speech Rehabilitation. Springfield, IL: Thomas, 1973.

10. Hirano M, Kuroiwa Y, Tanaka S, Matsuoka H, Sato K, Yoshida T. Dysphagia following various degrees of surgical resection for oral cancer. Ann Otol Rhinol Laryngol 1992;101:138–141.

11. Wheeler RL, Logemann JA, Rosen MS. Maxillary reshaping prosthesis: Effectiveness in improving speech and swallowing of post surgical oral cancer patients. J Prosthet Dent 1980;43:313–319.

12. Logemann JA, Kahrilas PJ, Hurst P, Davis J, Krugler C. Effects of intraoral prosthesis on swallowing in patients with oral cancer. Dysphagia 1989;4:118–120.

CHAPTER 17

Psychosocial Considerations

Victoria A. Wilson, MSW, LCSW-C

The impact of a cancer diagnosis on a patient and family cannot be overstated. When that diagnosis is oral cancer, the effects can be particularly devastating. In addition to the fear of death that all people face, the person with oral cancer faces unique, life-changing problems. Treatment modalities—surgery, radiation, and chemotherapy—can cause significant changes in appearance. Functions such as speech, taste, mastication, smell, the ability to swallow, and certain sexual behaviors may be altered. Self-image and stigmatization issues arise and require tremendous emotional strength on the part of the patient to integrate these changes into his or her life. Family members experience a parallel emotional process.

Throughout the continuum of the disease process (diagnosis, treatment, rehabilitation, possible recurrence, retreatment, possible death), it is normal to witness depression and anxiety. Suicidal ideation is not uncommon. Having an oral cancer, plus other risk factors such as poor prognosis and substance abuse history (often seen in this population), may increase the risk for suicidality.[1]

The patient who has used alcohol and tobacco must face emotions related to their role in the etiology of the cancer. A history of alcoholism may complicate medical management by poor compliance and nonadaptive coping strategies. Alcoholism also potentiates psychiatric problems. In a study by Regier et al,[2] 39% of alcoholics had a second psychiatric diagnosis. It is clear that the patient with a neoplasm of the oral cavity faces psychological problems and social stressors related to the cancer, treatment sequelae, and premorbid issues. This chapter explores the myriad psychosocial issues inherent in the oral cancer experience, the impact on psychological adjustment and rehabilitation, and specific insights and recommendations for interventions by physicians.

Psychological Reactions

Psychological investment in the head and neck area is greater than in any other part of the body because social interaction and emo-

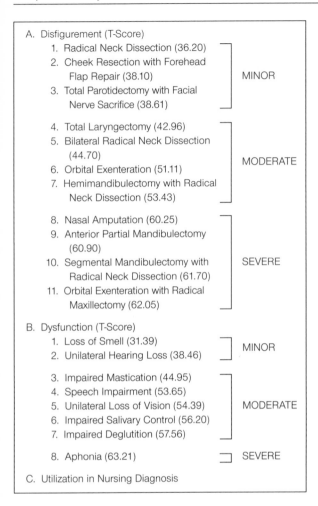

A. Disfigurement (T-Score)
  1. Radical Neck Dissection (36.20)
  2. Cheek Resection with Forehead
     Flap Repair (38.10)   MINOR
  3. Total Parotidectomy with Facial
     Nerve Sacrifice (38.61)

  4. Total Laryngectomy (42.96)
  5. Bilateral Radical Neck Dissection
     (44.70)   MODERATE
  6. Orbital Exenteration (51.11)
  7. Hemimandibulectomy with Radical
     Neck Dissection (53.43)

  8. Nasal Amputation (60.25)
  9. Anterior Partial Mandibulectomy
     (60.90)
  10. Segmental Mandibulectomy with   SEVERE
     Radical Neck Dissection (61.70)
  11. Orbital Exenteration with Radical
     Maxillectomy (62.05)

B. Dysfunction (T-Score)
  1. Loss of Smell (31.39)   MINOR
  2. Unilateral Hearing Loss (38.46)

  3. Impaired Mastication (44.95)
  4. Speech Impairment (53.65)
  5. Unilateral Loss of Vision (54.39)   MODERATE
  6. Impaired Salivary Control (56.20)
  7. Impaired Deglutition (57.56)

  8. Aphonia (63.21)   SEVERE

C. Utilization in Nursing Diagnosis

Fig 17-1   Disfigurement/dysfunction scale. Alteration in body image related to specific disfigurement or dysfunction as evidenced by disfigurement/dysfunction scale. (Reprinted by permission of John Wiley and Sons from Dropkin et al.[4])

tional expression depend to a great extent on the integrity of the face, especially the eyes.[3] Alterations in the oral cavity due to cancer and treatment can affect form and function; impairments can affect intimacy (affection and sexuality), communication (speech), and socialization (eating, occupation). It is not surprising that fears of isolation, stigmatization, and abandonment affect decisions about treatment, particularly surgery. Preoperatively, patients may experience high anxiety regarding anticipated functional and cosmetic losses. Postoperatively, patients may experience grief and depression related to their "lost" self. Dropkin and colleagues[4] developed a scale of

disfigurement and dysfunction to assist the medical team in postoperative care (Fig 17-1).

Many of the disfigurements and dysfunctions that patients experience postoperatively, such as segmental mandibulectomy with radical neck dissection, and speech, salivation, and mastication impairments, fall into the moderate to severe categories. In studies using the scale and the concept of a body reintegration model in predicting rehabilitation problems, more severe functional and/or structural loss was associated with slower recovery, more prolonged social isolation, lower self-esteem, greater sense of worthlessness, and more severe depression.[3] In a study[5] that examined the postoperative adjustment of patients who underwent surgery for cancers of the head and neck (18 [45%] had oral cavity or oropharyngeal cancers), it was found that patients undergoing radiation postoperatively tended to have greater difficulty adjusting to the disease and treatment, particularly when these were compounded by physical difficulties and financial stressors.

Patients with cancers of the oral cavity and oropharynx, as well as those who underwent composite surgical resections, found the postoperative period most difficult. Jenkins and colleagues[6] found that a personal or family history of treated depression, not the number of radiation treatments received, was predictive of those patients with depressive symptoms. There is a dearth of literature on the impact of oral cancer on sexuality and intimacy. However, this impact seems as clinically significant in patients with oral cancer as it is with patients who have undergone mastectomy and colostomy.[7] The correlation is clear: the greater the functional and cosmetic change, the greater the impact on self-image and level of emotional distress.

Case report

A 50-year-old married man in whom a stage III carcinoma of the tongue had recently been diagnosed was referred by the surgeon for presurgical counseling with an oncology social worker. The patient felt paralyzed by anxiety and had told the surgeon he wanted to cancel the surgery. Fears of loss of speech, the surgical procedure itself, death from cancer, loss of ability to work, and having a "nervous breakdown" were identified. The patient had experienced a nervous breakdown 2 years earlier and felt himself decompensating into this psychological state. The patient was given an opportunity to express his fears and emotions, speak with his surgeon regarding questions/concerns, and introduced to the medical floor and nursing staff. A description of other supportive services such as nutrition and speech therapy was offered. Introduction to a veteran patient with the same diagnosis and treatment interventions was offered but declined, as was a psychiatric consultation for psychotropic medication. The patient followed through with the surgical treatment plan and after an uneventful hospitalization, went home.

After discharge, the patient was again referred for counseling regarding a treatment decision: radiation therapy had been recommended due to lymph node involvement. The patient had strong negative images of radiation and its side effects. His decision after four counseling sessions was to not receive radiation therapy. Approximately 6 months later, a recurrence was found in the neck and the patient was again strongly advised by physicians to receive radiation. The patient reported a doctor saying "receive radiation or die." Even with this perspective, the patient struggled with the decision due to his fear of the side effects. After a few counseling sessions, the patient did agree to radiation therapy and was followed throughout treatment by the counselor. It was during this phase that the patient's fear about self-image, particularly his self-image concerning sexuality and attractiveness, was identified. Due to the partial glossectomy and reduced salivation, the patient was uncomfortable with oral intimacy. He moved out of the bedroom he shared with his wife as a way of coping. The patient terminated counseling soon after, when radiation therapy was completed.

This case reflects the value of counseling for a patient facing difficult treatment decisions and the impact of treatment sequelae on self-image and relationships. This patient used withdrawal as his coping strategy. If he had continued in counseling, finding more adaptive strategies would have been a paramount goal.

Table 17-1	Common Psychiatric Problems in Patients with Head and Neck Cancer
Problem areas	**Components***
Emotional reactions to diagnosis and surgery	Anxiety Depression Suicide risk
Preexisting personality and coping style	Unrelated to alcohol and tobacco use Related to alcohol and tobacco use
Alcohol and tobacco-related disorders	Alcoholism Alcohol withdrawal syndromes Delirium tremens Wernicke-Korsakoff's syndrome Alcohol-associated dementia Competency to sign consent forms Poor compliance Tobacco withdrawal syndrome
Rehabilitation	Difficulty adapting to structural change Delayed socialization Psychosocial concerns of rejection Psychosexual difficulties Difficulty adapting to dysfunction Self-care Use of prosthesis Use of artificial larynx Learning of esophageal speech Continued smoking and drinking

*Of the 23 components listed, all but the two related to laryngectomies (use of artificial larynx and learning of esophageal speech) affect the person with oral cancer.

Psychosocial Issues Related to Diagnosis and Treatment

Commonly seen psychological responses and psychiatric complications with head and neck cancer that require recognition and management are the emotional reactions to diagnosis and treatment, preexisting personality and coping style, alcohol- and tobacco-related disorders, and rehabilitation[3] (Table 17-1). Of the 23 components listed, all but the two related to laryngectomies (use of artificial larynx and learning of esophageal speech) affect the per-

son with oral cancer. Psychological issues begin at diagnosis. A diagnosis of cancer immediately brings up fear and a loss of control, which often manifest as anxiety, grief, and depression. These reactions are normal and adaptive up to a point, but it is important to monitor the intensity and duration. According to Goodwin,[8] patients with head and neck cancer, as a result of the appearance-altering surgery and frequent alcoholic history, have a higher risk of depression and suicide than the general cancer population. If the patient has a premorbid history or the symptoms interfere with the patient's ability to function in life, including participation in medical treatment, a psychotherapeutic intervention is indicated.

Preoperatively, a patient must face fears of the procedure itself and anticipated changes in function and apppearance. These fears can result in indecision about treatment choices and delay in the initiation of treatment. Rehabilitation should start during this phase with a preoperative psychosocial assessment, including a family and social history, coping strategies, intrapersonal and interpersonal resources, and alcohol and drug history. Introduction to medical team members, including a nurse, social worker, and speech language pathologist, ameliorates feelings of anxiety and isolation. It is important to educate the patient and family fully regarding the surgery itself, the hospital stay, and staff support, eg, discharge planning. The opportunity to meet with a veteran patient who has undergone similar treatment should be offered for information and support.

For those patients with high emotional distress, a premorbid psychiatric history, alcoholism and/or drug history, and a lack of interpersonal support, a referral for counseling with a psychotherapist who has a knowledge of medical issues should be made. During hospitalization, the patient is faced with physical recovery as well as changes in appearance. To lack the ability to speak or swallow, even temporarily, can be frightening. Pain reactions may increase anxiety and dependency on others (family and hospital personnel) and increase feelings of helplessness. Team members can help patients confront changes in their appearance by encouraging them to look in the mirror and being present with them if requested. It is important that this happen before discharge from the hospital. Dropkin et al[4] found that 5 days after surgery was the critical point in recovery in terms of acceptance of the defect, participation in self-care, and resocialization. When rehabilitation starts early in treatment, patients at risk of poor adaptation

can be identified and supports put in place as soon as possible.

The medical team often makes the mistake of assuming discharge is always a positive event. Leaving the womblike environment of the hospital where care is round the clock and a "button away" can actually increase feelings of anxiety and depression. To better support the patient and family through the discharge process, the medical team should validate the patient's ambivalence, address practical concerns such as home care and equipment, and schedule outpatient follow-up.

Throughout the continuum of care from diagnosis to death, the medical and dental team should be aware of the need for and benefits of supportive psychotherapy. It is important to normalize the "craziness" of the cancer experience: even people with intact ego integrity and positive family lives need emotional support during a cancer crisis.

Medical Crisis Counseling,[9] a model of brief counseling designed to support those living with a life-changing chronic illness, focuses on eight core issues that seem universal to the cancer experience (Table 17-2).

In counseling, the focus should be on giving the patient and/or family the opportunity to express their emotions and have their experience validated. The goal is one of integration: designing a quality life that includes the illness and sequelae. There may be times when supportive counseling alone is not enough. Approximately 20% to 35% of patients with cancer warrant evaluations for elevated emotional distress.[10] A psychiatric consultation may be indicated in the following situations: history of psychiatric problems, addiction history, refractory depression and anxiety, suicidal ideation, and assessment/treatment for psychotropic medications. Mood disorders among patients have been thoroughly researched, but the use of psychotropic medication in their management has not.[11]

Table 17-2	Medical Crisis Counseling
Core issues	Objective
Loss of control	To reestablish control
Loss of self-image	To grieve losses and redefine the self
Dependency	To combine maximum self-reliance with acceptance of a level of physical dependence
Stigma	To develop the self-acceptance and social skills needed to deal with others' attitudes
Abandonment	To be able to face difficult decisions with realism and sensitivity to others' needs
Anger	To identify and redirect anger, and thereby release constructive energy
Isolation	To sustain an appropriate level of meaningful contact with others
Death	To promote existential acceptance with an emphasis on the quality of life in the here and now

Case report

A 50-year-old white man with stage IV carcinoma of the floor of the mouth and tongue presented for counseling in July 1998, at the advice of his oral surgeon due to his increasing depressive symptoms and suicidal ideation. The diagnosis of oral cancer had been made in March 1997, followed by surgery that same month, radiation therapy in the summer of 1997, reparative surgery in September 1997, and bone graft surgery in March 1998. The patient felt his depression exacerbate in May 1998, when his doctor told him that his inability to swallow food would most likely be permanent. The patient was seen with his wife in the first session (only). He was experiencing feelings of hopelessness, angry outbursts, and fears of isolation and abandonment. He presented with the classic symptoms of depression, including suicidal

ideation. His wife had seen a therapist previously and was taking an antidepressant. The decision was made that the patient would participate in individual counseling. The patient was referred by the counselor to a psychiatrist for a medication consultation and was placed on an antidepressant in the form of a selective serotonin-reuptake inhibitor (SSRI).

He began Medical Crisis Counseling to explore issues concerning the cancer, treatment and sequelae, emotions and coping skills, and family relationships. The core issue of living with a life-changing and possibly terminal illness was the focus of therapy. The patient's primary concerns were his dysphasia, changes in his sexual drive and performance, and the inability to eat solids. Even after the patient's mood improved, his sexual self-image was such that he avoided physical intimacy. This was related to his impaired ability to use his lips and tongue or to feel sensation (due to postsurgical paresthesia). As the patient put it, "some men's sex life resides below the belt . . . mine resided above."

In addition to his struggle with self-image, his lack of sexual drive was exacerbated by the SSRI. The patient had had such a positive response to his medication in terms of his depressive symptoms that he did not want to change medications. Subsequent interventions included refining the dosage of the SSRI, using various medicines (including Viagra) to counteract the sexual side effects, and continued counseling. All the patient's symptoms of depression improved: increased energy and interest, better sleep, less withdrawal, less anxiety, and less rumination were noted. The suicidal ideation became an occasional existential question ("Is my life good enough to continue?") rather than an active, daily consideration of killing himself. Both his emotional and sexual relationships with his wife improved.

Issues Related to Alcohol and Tobacco

Many oral cancers occur in people with a history of excessive tobacco and alcohol use. In addition to the causative role, for which patients often feel guilt and regret, a substance abuse history poses additional problems. Among individuals who have abused alcohol and cigarettes before the development of head and neck cancer, personality characteristics of dependence, inability to change habits, and poor adaptive coping skills contribute to poor outcome.[3]

Excessive alcohol use often prompts disruption in the marriage and family, which can reduce social support. Struggles with work performance, finances, and legal issues may be present. Often alcohol and tobacco act as the person's primary coping strategy. At the most stressful time of the patient's life, the resource that has been used to sustain him or her is forbidden. Psychologically, this is very difficult. Poor physical health issues associated with alcoholism such as malnutrition and cirrhosis may be present, which may lead to impaired healing and special monitoring. Acute alcoholic withdrawal may result from hospitalization; postoperatively, delirium tremens may develop.

Usually, at the time of diagnosis, patients who smoke are told to stop. Surgery and hospitalization require it. Symptoms of tobacco withdrawal include anxiety, headache, irritability, agitation, sleep disturbance, impaired concentration and memory, and a craving for tobacco. Psychologically, the withdrawal of tobacco as a coping tool is likely to result in greater anxiety and distress. Substitute strategies should be considered, such as a referral to a smoking cessation group at the time of diagnosis, use of a nicotine patch, antianxiety medication, and relaxation/imagery techniques to minimize withdrawal symptoms.

Predictors of Psychological Distress

Weisman and Worden[12] report that only 40% to 60% of the variance associated with psychological distress is explained by purely medical factors. When looking at the prognostic signs of psychological adjustment, optimism regarding treatment, no history of psychiatric treatment, fewer marital problems before the diagnosis of cancer, higher socioeconomic status, less alcohol abuse, fewer physical symptoms associated with the disease, less advanced staging, and a coping strategy of finding something positive in the diagnostic situation were associated with lower emotional distress. Other factors affecting the level of distress and coping are degree of social isolation; history of recent loss (death, divorce); inflexible coping style; age; previous personal experiences with cancer; amount of change in appearance and function, especially speech; level of vocational support; perception of lack of family support; phase of illness and treatment; and importance of physical appearance and communication skills to self-image.

These factors affect treatment and psychological adaptation in various ways. For instance, a patient with a negative conceptualization of cancer and treatment, perhaps having lost a loved one to cancer, may delay seeking treatment, have more fear, resist treatment interventions, and be fatalistic regarding outcomes. A patient who is isolated and without social support is at higher psychological risk. A number of studies show that social support, which may manifest concretely (eg, assistance in the home, transportation, financial assistance) or as emotional support, can reduce the negative impact of illness and help to alleviate emotional distress.[13]

The availability of interpersonal support from family and loved ones is important at this time. The strain of dealing with the cancer and side effects can stress a relationship. Changes in appearance and the inability to maintain preexisting roles and functions may stress already strained relationships with loved ones and colleagues. The patient's premorbid personality traits and coping style play a large part in how relationships are maintained under duress. Patients with a history of positive relationships with family members, a network of family, and a good vocational history can be expected to be at lower risk of significant emotional distress.[14]

Awareness for patients' needs should be present during the entire illness continuum, but special attention should be paid at certain critical times. One investigation found that the period immediately after diagnosis was more emotionally stressful, as measured by self-reporting instruments, than the subsequent treatment period.[15] This may be due to the feelings of shock and fear that arise, a loss of control over one's body, and the loss of one's denial of mortality. With a recurrence, patients and families often feel a sense of hopelessness and realize that the odds of surviving the disease are lower. A feeling of hopelessness is overwhelming and has been shown to be an even stronger factor in predicting suicide than depression.[1]

If the cancer is deemed incurable, the medical team's support becomes paramount. The patient may want to continue treatment (eg, radiation therapy or surgery to reduce tumor burden) to gain time, lessen symptoms, and improve quality of life. A patient with head and neck cancer cannot be abandoned at the time when the need is greatest to have a constancy of physician presence.[16] By offering honest and clear communication, medical and emotional support, and referral for needed resources, medical providers influence in a positive way the patient's and family's ability to cope during this time and to mourn their losses.

Psychosocial Interventions

All interventions should begin with effective communication. Only by allowing the patient and family to articulate their needs can the doctor and team facilitate needed interventions. As previously stated, the concept of rehabilitation begins at diagnosis and continues through the illness process, even until death. The goal is not only to minimize emotional distress, but also to aid the patient and family in actively pursuing recovery and integrating the illness and sequelae into their lives. Members of the medical and dental team are critical players in terms of support and interventions as the patient defines what he or she sees as "quality of life." It is usually the surgeon who becomes the primary physician, the "quarterback" who calls the plays and leads the team members. The surgeon should have an effective team in place: radiation and medical oncologists, internists, restorative dentists and prosthodontists, speech/swallowing therapists, social workers, nutritionists, psychologists, and psychiatrists. With so many caregivers, it is necessary that the primary physician take on the pivotal role of maintaining communication and coordinating specialty care.

Physician-Patient Communication

Patients are much more aware of their doctor's ability to communicate with them effectively than with their technical expertise. In fact, patients' dissatisfaction with their physician's communication skills often far outweighs any dissatisfaction with technical competence.[17] Mistakes made in communicating to patients and families include:

- Not allowing enough time, thus appearing rushed or disinterested.
- Using medical jargon, which is confusing and may sound patronizing.
- Being a poor listener and not allowing the patient to talk.
- Using a detached verbal or physical stance as a way of "managing" emotion (this comes across as uncaring).
- Talking down to the patient.
- Projecting one's own needs and values onto the patient.
- Giving up on the need to communicate if the disease becomes terminal. This can occur out of a sense of failure and impotency on the doctor's part; the patient feels dehumanized and abandoned.

Checking in with patients regarding the amount of information they wish to have is the first step. The need to know or not know is very individualistic. Patients' personalities and coping styles vary, as do their reactions to information. For one patient, detailed information gives a feeling of being educated and in control; for another, that much information may feel overwhelming and be anxiety producing. The only way the doctor will know is by listening. With regard to giving bad news related to diagnosis, treatment, and prognosis, the physician should take the lead from the patient, who will either ask directly or give cues as to how much he or she wants to know.

In a study by Strauss,[18] 28 patients who had disfiguring oral and maxillofacial surgery for head and neck cancer were interviewed regarding the interpersonal and social ramifications of diagnosis and surgical treatment. Of the 21 patients (75%) who were able to share thoughts about death, 12 (43%) indicated that they could have benefited from more discussions with their surgeons about their chances of dying. The doctor should say, "How much information do you want? I am open and want to share information in a way that works best for you." To be open, empathic, and active in the communication process requires self-knowledge on the part of the provider. In this situation, "physician, know thyself" is imperative.

In the patient with an oral neoplasm, the major psychosocial issues revolve around practical needs related to functional changes and emotional reactions to the "lost self." Based on a complete psychosocial assessment, referrals should be considered (Table 17-3).

A systematic evaluation of a patient's intrapersonal and interpersonal resources should begin with diagnosis and continue through the treatment. Linking the patient to the appropriate resources as soon as possible minimizes anxiety, enables the patient to function at as high a capacity as possible, and fosters a sense

Table 17–3   Possible Referrals Based on Patient Need

Need	Discipline
Assessment and counseling: individual, family, couple, group, sexual, addiction	Therapist; eg, social worker, psychiatrist, psychologist
Financial, vocational problems	Social worker
Speech and swallowing therapy	Speech therapist
Psychotrophic medications	Psychiatrist
Referral to community resources; eg, support groups, American Cancer Society, funding for augmentative communication devices, etc	Social worker, speech language pathologist, nurse
Dental reconstruction	General dentist, prosthodontist
Educational programs	Social worker, nurse
Dietary	Nutritionist
Spiritual support	Hospital chaplain, clergy of patient's choice

of caring and support between physician and patient. Most patients, with the appropriate help, can lead full and productive lives.

Summary

Patients with a diagnosis of oral cancer face crises on many different levels: physical, spiritual, psychological, vocational, financial, social, sexual, and existential. Treatment options—surgery, radiation, and chemotherapy—often offer the possibility of cure, but sometimes at an overwhelming cost of loss of form, function, and appearance. Certain issues, such as premorbid personality traits, addiction, lack of social support, and psychiatric history, influence a patient's ability to cope and require increased advocacy on his or her behalf. All patients should be assessed as early as possible in the treatment process so that appropriate professional caregivers and resources may be used.

The goal of treatment should be, from the time of diagnosis to termination of treatment or life, to help the patient and family adapt to the changes brought on by oral cancer and to maximize the quality of their daily lives.

References

1. Henderson JM, Ord RA. Suicide in head and neck cancer patients. J Oral Maxillofac Surg 1997;55:1217–1221.

2. Regier DA, Farmer ME, Rae DS, et al. Co-morbidity of mental disorders with alcohol and other drug abuse. Results from the Epidemiologic Catchment Area (ECA) study. JAMA 1990;264:2511–2518.

3. Breitbart W, Holland JC. Head and neck cancer. In: Holland JC, Rainland JH (eds). Handbook of Psychooncology. New York: Oxford University Press, 1989:232–239.

4. Dropkin MJ, Malgady RK, Scott DW, Oberst M, Strong EW. Scaling of disfigurement and dysfunction in postoperative head and neck patients. Head Neck Surg 1983;8:559–570.

5. Krouse J, Krouse HJ, Fabian RL. Adaptation to surgery for head and neck cancer. Laryngoscope 1989;99: 789–794.

6. Jenkins C, Carmody T, Rush SJ. Depression in radiation oncology patients: A preliminary evaluation. J Affective Disord 1998;50:17–21.

7. Curtis TA, Zlatolow IM. Sexuality and head and neck cancer. Front Radiat Ther Oncol 1980;14:26–34.

8. Goodwin DW. Alcoholism and suicide. In: Patism EM, Kaufman E (eds). The Encyclopedia Handbook of Alcoholism. New York: Gardner Press, 1982:655–662.

9. Pollin I. Medical Crisis Counseling: Short-Term Therapy for Long-Term Illness. New York: Norton, 1995:47–92.

10. Stefanik ME. Psychosocial issues of head and neck cancer. In: Eisle DW (ed). Complications in Head and Neck Surgery. St Louis: Mosby, 1993:164–170.

11. Hughes J. Anxiety and depression: Psychotropic medication. In: Cancer Patient Care: Psychosocial Treatment Methods. Cambridge: Cambridge University Press, 1991:111–125.

12. Weisman A, Worden J. Coping and vulnerability in cancer patients. Boston: Project Omega, Harvard Medical School, Massachusetts General Hospital, 1976.

13. Rowland JH. Intrapersonal resources: Coping. In: Holland JC, Rowland JH (eds). Handbook of Psychooncology. New York: Oxford University Press, 1989:44–57.

14. Goldberg RT. Vocational and social adjustment after laryngectomy. Scand J Rehabil Med 1975;7:1–8.

15. Manual GM, Roth S, Keefe FJ, Brantley BA. Coping with cancer. J Human Stress 1987;4:149–158.

16. Roa RA, Eisele DW. Care of the patient with incurable head and neck cancer. In: Eisele DW (ed). Complications in Head and Neck Surgery. St Louis: Mosby, 1993:171–173.

17. Ben-Sira Z. The function of the professional's affective behavior in client satisfaction. J Health Soc Behav 1976;17:3–11.

18. Strauss RP. Psychosocial responses to oral and maxillofacial surgery for head and neck cancer. J Oral Maxillofac Surg 1989;47:343–348.

PART IV

Prevention

CHAPTER 18

Tobacco Cessation: The Dentist's Challenge

Jacquelyn L. Fried, RDH, MS

It is a fact that tobacco use has a causal relationship with the incidence of oral cancer. Regardless of tobacco's mode of delivery— smokeless tobacco (ST), cigarettes, cigars, or pipes—its use has carcinogenic potential.[1,2] Tobacco use overall is implicated in 75% of oral and pharyngeal cancers,[3] while scientific reports have established that ST use can cause oral cancer.[4] It has been reported that in long-term snuff users, oral cancer may occur in certain sites as much as 50 times more frequently than among nonusers.[5]

Despite the fact that the American public is inundated with information stating the ill effects of tobacco use, approximately 25% of the population continues to smoke cigarettes.[6] Another 12 million Americans routinely use ST,[4] while cigar sales have increased by almost 50% since 1993.[7] Over 400,000 Americans die annually from tobacco-related illnesses,[8] yet these illnesses, including oral cancers, are among the most preventable types of disease.[9]

The National Cancer Institute (NCI), in its efforts to stem the incidence of cancer, has vigorously endorsed and promoted the role of the dentist, the dental hygienist, and the entire oral health team in aiding tobacco-using patients in their efforts to abstain.[9] Oral health care professionals also have been charged with preventing the initiation of tobacco use among youth in the United States.[9] Under the auspices of both the NCI and the Agency for Health Care Policy and Research (AHCPR), the clinical roles of oral health care professionals have been designated, delineated, described, and scientifically studied.[9,10] Healthy People 2000 includes 26 objectives that encompass the tobacco priority area. Specifically, objective 3.16 proposes to "Increase to at least 75% (by the year 2000) the proportion of primary care and oral health care providers who routinely advise cessation and provide assistance and follow-up for all of their tobacco-using patients."[11]

Recent surveys reveal that the number of oral health care providers actively engaged in tobacco interventions, although improving, still falls short of the Healthy People 2000's benchmark. In their 1996 study, Tomar et al[12] reported that fewer than one fourth of smokers reported that they had been advised by their dentists to quit smoking during the previous year, while 51% claimed to have been so advised by their physicians. Dolan et al,[13] in a more recent publication, looked at specific tobacco use intervention behaviors among a national sample of dentists and dental hygienists. The results revealed that less than one third of dentists or dental hygienists provided any cessation services for patients. Typically, the respondents routinely did not ask about tobacco use or document tobacco use status in the patient's record. If they knew that patients were users, they were likely to advise them to quit but not as likely to provide services to help them stop.

In the study by Dolan et al,[13] about half of the subjects claimed that lack of insurance reimbursement, not knowing where to send the patient for counseling, lack of confidence, and the amount of time required were barriers to providing tobacco cessation services to patients. In their study of Maryland dentists, Fried and Cohen[14] found that a perceived lack of knowledge and skill deterred many dentists from actively engaging in tobacco use intervention behaviors; however, respondents also expressed an interest in obtaining skills training in this area. Clinical trials have shown that dentists can be highly effective in delivering brief yet effective tobacco intervention messages, and 1-year quit rates as high as 15% have been reported in dentist-initiated endeavors.[15]

Oral health care providers represent an important group of clinicians who can be instrumental in waging war on tobacco use and its associated effects. More than 50% of US smokers see their dentists at least once a year[12,16]; therefore, a population in need of tobacco intervention services is readily available. Dental practices provide an ideal tobacco use intervention environment. Many appointments are "well visits" in that patients present for preventive maintenance; their nonemergency status may facilitate intervention efforts. Also, patients often have multiple visits and/or are on a regular recall schedule.

Messages may then be reinforced and patients observed. Oral health care practitioners also are provided "the teachable moment":[17] oral effects of tobacco use are visible in the patient's mouth, so the ramifications of tobacco use can be shown to the patient and can serve as a strong impetus to cessation.

On a daily basis, dentists use many of the skills essential to tobacco use intervention activities. Communications that explain, inform, influence, and motivate patients are typically used in everyday practice. Dentists possess an arsenal of information related to health behaviors, oral pathosis, and patient compliance, just to name a few. Dentists also know their patients well, are trusted by them, and have their respect. These combined strengths automatically give dentists an advantage in their assumption of tobacco intervention roles. Finally, prevention and education are hallmarks of successful dental practices. Practices with a holistic bent that are concerned with the overall well-being of the patient represent the highest level of professional ethics dentistry can offer. It has been suggested that monitoring the tobacco use habits of dental patients is as critical as monitoring other key vital signs, such as blood pressure.[18] Others state that the inclusion of tobacco use intervention activities in primary care practices needs to become an expected standard of care[19,20] and may be an essential risk management activity.[21] In the anticipated revision of the American Dental Association's (ADA's) health history form, additional questions addressing the patient's tobacco use history will be included.[19] The ADA already has an insurance code (no. 01320) designated for "Tobacco Counseling for the Prevention and Control of Oral Disease."

All of the aforementioned developments highlight the dentist's recognized and affirmed role in tobacco use prevention and cessation activities. Dentists have key responsibilities as role models, authorities, and educators in informing the public about the dangers of tobacco use.[9,13,14,19] They must personally aid their patients in cessation efforts.

This chapter is designed to assist the practicing dentist in comfortably assuming the role of tobacco use interventionist. The highlighted interventions stress brief yet effective behaviors that are science based and have proven to be successful in clinical dental settings.[9,10] Useful approaches that enhance patient success are explored and a discussion of pharmacologic adjuncts in the cessation process is included.

After reading this material, it is hoped that dental providers will possess the requisite knowledge, confidence, and motivation to incorporate tobacco use intervention behaviors into their daily practices. Assumption of these behaviors can promise increased personal and professional satisfaction, gratified patients who may serve as future referral sources, more positive treatment outcomes, and, most importantly, the opportunity to prevent disease and save lives.

The framework for the following text is based on the AHCPR clinical practice guideline for smoking cessation[10] and is supported by documents developed by the National Cancer Institute.[9] The AHCPR clinical strategies (Table 18-1) embody the NCI 4 As protocol of Ask, Advise, Assist, and Arrange.

The Clinic/Practice Environment

Before introducing the demonstrable behaviors that comprise effective tobacco use interventions, a word about the overall office atmosphere is necessary. For a tobacco use intervention program to be successful, the total dental practice environment must convey an atmosphere of commitment and support. Team members need to endorse the philosophy of a tobacco-free staff, patient population, and office environment. In their interactions with patients, the dentist and all team members must be knowledgeable about the tobacco intervention process and supportive of patient efforts. The more reinforcement patients receive, the greater their chances for success.[10] Team members who work with patients using the 4 As must document all patient efforts in the chart and stay abreast of patient progress. An office-specific "tickler" system can ensure that patients are monitored. Material available from the AHCPR[10] can direct practice protocol; staff meetings and in-service sessions designed to educate team members about the office tobacco use intervention program also will facilitate team endorsement and the timely implementation of a tobacco intervention program.

The dentist also should designate a team coordinator (eg, the dental hygienist or dental assistant) to oversee program activities.[9] This individual should be committed, enthusiastic, and organized. The coordinator ensures that all team members fully understand the intervention program and can plan in-service activities to achieve this end. The coordinator also monitors patient and program progress and offers recommendations for improvement. The key point is that someone on the dental team must be responsible for the effective implementation of the tobacco use intervention program.

The physical office environment can convey a commitment to tobacco use interventions through the procurement and display of relevant patient literature. The creation of a congratulatory "I quit" bulletin board or the inclusion of tobacco prevention information in office newsletters are other ways. The availability of patient education materials is boundless; literature can be obtained at no

Table 18-1   AHCPR Strategies

Strategy 1. Ask—systematically identify all tobacco users at every visit

Action	Strategies for implementation
Implement an office-wide system that ensures that, for *every* patient at *every* clinic visit, tobacco-use status is queried and documented.*	Expand the vital signs to include tobacco use. • Data collected by health care team. • Implemented using preprinted progress note paper that includes the expanded vital signs, a vital signs stamp, or, for computerized records, includes an item assessing tobacco-use status.

VITAL SIGNS

Blood Pressure: _____

Pulse: _____   Weight: _____

Temperature: _____

Respiratory Rate: _____

Tobacco Use (circle one):   Current   Former   Never

Alternatives to the vital signs stamp are to place tobacco-use status stickers on all patient charts or to indicate smoking status using computer reminder systems.

*Repeated assessment is not necessary in the case of the adult who has never smoked or not smoked for many years, and for whom this information is clearly documented in the medical record.

Strategy 2. Advise—strongly urge all smokers to quit

Action	Strategies for implementation
In a *clear, strong,* and *personalized* manner, urge every smoker to quit.	Advice should be: • Clear — "I think it is important for you to quit smoking now and I will help you." "Cutting down while you are ill is not enough." • Strong — "As your clinician, I need you to know that quitting smoking is the most important thing you can do to protect your current and future health." • Personalized — Tie smoking to current health/illness, and/or the social and economic costs of tobacco use, motivation level/readiness to quit, and/or the impact of smoking on children and others in the household. Encourage clinic staff to reinforce the cessation message and support the patient's quit attempt.

Strategy 3. Identify smokers willing to make a quit attempt

Action	Strategies for implementation
Ask every smoker if he or she is willing to make a quit attempt at this time.	• If the patient is willing to make a quit attempt at this time, provide assistance. • If the patient prefers a more intensive treatment or the clinician believes intensive treatment is appropriate, refer to interventions administered by a smoking cessation specialist and follow up with the patient regarding quitting. • If the patient clearly states he/she is not willing to make a quit attempt at this time, provide a motivational intervention. Also, if the patient is a member of a special population (eg, adolescent, pregnant smoker, racial/ethnic minority), additional information is available from AHCPR.

Table 18-1   AHCPR Strategies (Continued)

Strategy 4.   Assist—aid the patient in quitting

Action	Strategies for implementation
Help the patient with a quit plan.	Set a quit date—Ideally, the quit date should be within 2 weeks, taking patient preference into account.
	A patient's preparations for quitting:
	• Inform family, friends, and coworkers of quitting and request understanding and support.
	• Remove cigarettes from your environment. Prior to quitting, avoid smoking in places where you spend a lot of time (eg, home, car).
	• Review previous quit attempts. What helped you? What led to relapse?
	• Anticipate challenges to planned quit attempt, particularly during the critical first few weeks. These include nicotine withdrawal symptoms.
Encourage nicotine replacement therapy except in special circumstances.	Encourage the use of nicotine patch or nicotine gum therapy for smoking cessation.
Give key advice on successful quitting.	Abstinence—Total abstinence is essential. "Not even a single puff after the quit date."
	Alcohol—Drinking alcohol is highly associated with relapse. Those who stop smoking should review their alcohol use and consider limiting/abstaining from alcohol during the quit process.
	Other smokers in the household—The presence of other smokers in the household, particularly a spouse, is associated with lower success rates. Patients should consider quitting with their significant others and/or developing specific plans to stay quit in a household where others still smoke.
Provide supplementary materials.	Sources—Federal agencies, including AHCPR; nonprofit agencies (ACS, ALA, AHA); or local/state health departments.
	Type—Culturally/racially/educationally/age appropriate for the patient.
	Location—Readily available in every clinic office.

Strategy 5.   Arrange—schedule follow-up contact

Action	Strategies for implementation
Schedule follow-up contact, either in person or via telephone.	Timing—Follow-up contact should occur soon after the quit date, preferably during the first week. A second follow-up contact is recommended within the first month. Schedule further follow-up contacts as indicated.
	Action during follow-up visit—Congratulate success. If smoking occurred, review circumstances and elicit recommitment to total abstinence. Remind patient that a lapse can be used as a learning experience. Identify problems already encountered and anticipate challenges in the immediate future. Assess nicotine replacement therapy use and problems. Consider referral to a more intense or specialized program.

Adapted from AHCPR Publication No. 96-0692, US Department of Health and Human Services, April 1996, pp 22–25.

cost from the federal government or for low cost from local nonprofit organizations (eg, the American Cancer Society, the American Lung Association). The American Dental Hygienists' Association (1-800-243-2322) and American Dental Association (1-800-621-8099) also offer tobacco-related materials for sale through their catalogues.

In summary, a practice-based tobacco use intervention program is only as strong as the team that supports it and makes it work on a daily basis.[9] As key leaders of the practice, dentists need to convey strong statements of support for tobacco use intervention; in turn, the rest of the team will more readily claim ownership of an endeavor that can bring new life and challenge to a practice.

Step-by-Step Strategies

Strategy 1. Ask

A key phrase in today's world of dentistry is "risk assessment." To establish a patient's risk for oral cancer, the dental provider needs to be aware of the patient's tobacco use status and of any other deleterious contributing factors. Thus, the first strategy in any tobacco use intervention is identifying the tobacco-using patient. This occurs during the Ask phase of the patient assessment. All patients at every clinic visit must be asked about their tobacco use status and their responses must be documented. An officewide system must ensure that this action takes place. The patient's tobacco use status can be ascertained most easily through patient completion of a health history form. If the current health history form does not include questions relating to tobacco use, the patient needs to be asked. Questions addressing use status (eg, current,

former, never), extent and duration of use, type of tobacco used, and previous quit attempts should be included in all queries whether obtained verbally or through health history questionnaires. Information that goes beyond just knowing whether the patient is a current user assists the dentist in risk assessment, because greater exposure and length of use correlate with increased disease incidence.[2,9,10] Clearly, patients who use any tobacco in any form are at higher risk for oral cancer than their nonusing or formerly using counterparts. In addition, the type of tobacco used may shape intervention efforts and help direct intraoral and extraoral examinations. Other relevant information about a patient's social history that should be obtained during the Ask phase relates to alcohol consumption and exposure to sun.[22] Alcohol has a synergistic effect with tobacco and may increase a patient's risk for oral cancer.[23-25] Similarly, sun exposure is a risk factor for lip cancers.[26] Knowing the extent of patient exposure to these variables helps the dentist further assess risk. Questions addressing these issues may be included in a health history form or added to a tobacco use assessment form (Fig 18-1).

For successful implementation of the Advising and Assisting strategies of the AHCPR clinical practice guideline, an understanding of why patients begin and sustain the tobacco use habit is helpful. Why do individuals initiate tobacco use? What drives their decision? Although these questions have no easy answers, some insights are offered. First, most smokers establish their habit during adolescence; in fact, over 89% of long-term users report having started by age 18.[27] Adolescence is marked by experimentation, risk-taking, and the search for identity. The feeling of indomitability coupled with sophisticated and targeted tobacco advertising makes the young teenager vulnerable to tobacco's attraction.[27,28] Sports figures, movie

---

Tobacco Use Assessment Form

Name _____   Date _____

1. Do you use tobacco in any form?   Yes _____ No _____

1A. If no, have you ever used tobacco in the past?   Yes _____ No _____

How long did you use tobacco?   Years _____ Months _____
How long ago did you stop?   Years _____ Months _____

If you are not currently a tobacco user, no other questions should be answered.
Thank you for completing this form.

Questions 2-10 are for current tobacco users only.

2. If you smoke, what type? (Check)   How many? (Number)

      Cigarettes _____   Cigarettes per day _____
      Cigars _____   Cigars per day _____
      Pipe _____   Bowls per day _____

3. If you chew/use snuff, what type?   How much?

      Snuff _____   days a can lasts _____
      Chewing _____   pouches per week _____
      Other (describe) _____   amount _____ per _____

3A. How long do you keep a chew in your mouth?   Minutes _____

4. How many days of the week do you use tobacco?   7 6 5 4 3 2 1

5. How soon after you wake up do you first use tobacco?   Within 30 minutes _____
                                                 More than 30 minutes _____

6. Does the person closest to you use tobacco?   Yes _____ No _____

7. How interested are you in stopping your use of tobacco?

     Not at all _____   A little _____   Somewhat _____   Very much _____

8. Have you tried to stop using tobacco before?   Yes _____ No _____

8A. How long ago was your last try to stop?   Years _____ Months _____

9. Have you discussed stopping with your physician?   Yes _____ No _____

10. If you decided to stop using tobacco completely during the next two weeks, how confident are
    you that you would succeed?
     Not at all _____   A little _____   Somewhat _____   Very confident _____

Fig 18-1 The Tobacco Use Assessment Form can be used to document patient tobacco use information and to direct intervention activities.[2]

stars, and models who use and glamorize tobacco further mislead young individuals. The tobacco industry promotes the use of "starter products," and confectioners manufacture items that mimic tobacco products, such as candy cigarettes and bubblegum rolled in a tin. All these factors lure young people into habituation and maintenance.[27]

Once individuals initiate and become comfortable with their habits, the physiologic addiction to nicotine follows.[29] Nicotine dependence can be considered a brain disease embedded in a social context.[19] Social and psychological factors complete the constellation of dependencies that impact the tobacco-using patient.[9] For example, women who smoke cigarettes fear weight gain if they abstain, so socially their habit is reinforced.[30,31] Young male athletes may believe that the use of ST increases their athletic performance because many star athletes are users.[4] The complexity of the tobacco use habit reinforces the need for multiple intervention strategies, including behavioral support, the use of FDA-approved pharmacologic adjuncts, and possible referral to a more intense or specialized program.

Strategy 2. Advise

The second strategy in the intervention process is to Advise the patient to stop. Advising may be the most critical step in promoting patient receptivity. How the patient is advised can determine whether he or she is responsive, personally affronted, or cornered into denial. The Advise message must be clear, strong, and personalized. An understanding of the patient's habit also can lend empathy to the message. It is a challenge to advise skillfully.

Once tobacco-using patients have been identified, they must be advised to abstain. This message of abstinence must be stated firmly and unequivocally, yet caringly. Many practitioners fear offending their patients during the Advise phase. The key to success is ensuring that warmth and caring are implicit in the message.

Another important element of advising is personalization. Information obtained from the patient's health history and clinical and radiographic examinations can help drive the advising session. The oral effects of tobacco use must be shown to the patient. Related systemic issues also should be correlated with tobacco use. Radiographs that reveal extensive bone loss due to periodontal disease also personalize the message.

Strategy 3. Identify Smokers Willing to Make a Quit Attempt

The patient's desire to abstain must be ascertained before appropriate assistance can be offered. Not all patients will be willing, motivated, or committed to abstain at the initial encounter or even at several thereafter. For patients not willing to commit, the clinician should provide a brief motivational intervention. Patients not yet ready may be uninformed, concerned about the effects of quitting, or demoralized due to previous discouraging attempts. Whatever their reasons, these patients need supportive messages and systematic follow-up.

To help motivate patients, the dentist's message should include four key elements: relevance, risks, rewards, and repetition. These four Rs personalize the message to the patient by showing how tobacco use is relevant to the patient's life (eg, children in the home), what personal risks it incurs (eg, oral cancer), the rewards of abstinence (eg, less fear of oral cancer), and repetition (ie, the practitioner must

Table 18-2   FDA-Approved Pharmaceutical Agents

Replacement agent	Trade name	Manufacturer
Nicotine transdermal patch:		
21-14-7 mg	Nicoderm CQ (OTC)	SmithKline Beecham
21-14-7 mg	Habitrol	Ciba
22-11 mg	Prostep	Lederle
15 (10-5) mg	Nicotrol (OTC)	McNeil
Nicotine polacrilex (gum):		
2–4 mg	Nicorette (OTC)	SmithKline Beecham
Nicotine nasal spray:		
0.5 mg per squirt	Nicotrol NS	McNeil
Nicotine oral inhaler:		
2–2.5 mg in vapor	Nicotrol Inhaler	McNeil
Nonnicotine agent and dose:		
Buproprion HCl tablet:		
150 mg/day x 3 days, then 150 mg bid	Zyban	Glaxo-Wellcome

repeat these motivational messages). Because dentists are used to high levels of practice success, they must understand that behavioral change is incremental and often slow. However, the practitioner's motivational message may activate a series of thought processes in the patient that will result in the decision to abstain.

Strategy 4. Assist

For patients ready to abstain, a formalized game plan needs to be developed. This includes setting a "quit" date, preferably within the following 2 weeks; eliminating triggers to tobacco use from the immediate environment; requesting support and understanding from significant others; reviewing factors that helped or hampered previous quit attempts; and anticipating current challenges to the planned quit attempt. The plan needs to be individualized and orchestrated by the patient (eg, the patient should select the quit date). The provider's main roles are facilitative and

encouraging. The practitioner fosters success by giving key advice, reinforcing total abstinence, suggesting ways to deal with users living in the household, and providing supplemental patient-specific literature.

Another component of the Assist strategy is the use of FDA-approved pharmacologic adjuncts, both nicotine and nonnicotine (Table 18-2). Controlled clinical trials reveal that the use of nicotine replacement therapies (ie, the nicotine patch and nicotine gum) when compared with placebo and when used in conjunction with recommended behavioral interventions can significantly increase the rates of abstinence.[9,18]

Based on meta-analyses of multiple clinical trials, the AHCPR guidelines[10] strongly recommend the use of nicotine replacement therapy to support cessation efforts. Nicotine replacement products allow patients to wean themselves from the physiologic dependency of nicotine and are effective in reducing withdrawal symptoms. The use of any tobacco product is prohibited when patients are on nicotine replacement therapy.

The most researched nicotine replacement therapies are nicotine transdermal patches and nicotine gum. Due to its ease of use and high level of patient compliance, the nicotine patch may be the most acceptable modality across diverse populations. Its use can approximately double long-term quit rates.[10,19] Pregnant patients, patients with contraindicating cardiovascular disease (eg, serious arrhythmia), and those who experience severe skin reactions should be assessed thoroughly prior to use of the patch.

In studies with nicotine gum, investigators have reported problems with ease of use, compliance, social acceptability, and unpleasant taste. However, nicotine gum may be the mode of choice for select patients. In highly dependent smokers, the 4-mg gum has proved more efficacious than the 2-mg gum.[32] Specific dosages and instructions are needed to aid the patient with compliance.

Other nicotine-containing adjuncts that recently have received FDA approval include the nicotine nasal spray and the nicotine inhaler.[19] Published data on these products are limited, but their use does show promise in cessation efforts, especially when compared with placebo interventions. Specific instructions for use can be obtained from the manufacturers (see Table 18-2).

Although certain nicotine replacement therapies are over-the-counter, the availability of these products to patients does not diminish the dentist's interventional role. Dentists must still encourage over-the-counter product use when appropriate, provide instructions for proper usage, and offer supportive counseling. Patient use of non-over-the-counter approved nicotine replacement therapies (eg, select patches, nasal spray, inhaler) still requires a prescription, and the suitability of these therapies for patient usage requires the dentist's supervision and support.

A recently approved nonnicotine replacement therapy has been shown effective in countering nicotine reward and withdrawal effects in patients who smoke.[19] Buproprion hydrochloride (Zyban) may be an alternative for patients who have not succeeded when using nicotine replacement therapy or who have experienced excessive weight gain with previous attempts.[33]

The appropriate selection and use of ADA-approved nicotine and nonnicotine pharmacologic adjuncts require the dentist's sound professional judgment. Patient success rests with careful decision making, instruction, and monitoring. More specific product information may be obtained from the manufacturers as well as from the ADA Guide to Dental Therapeutics, first edition, available from the American Dental Association (1-800-621-8099).

Strategy 5. Arrange

Arranging follow-up is crucial to successful cessation efforts. Patients must be contacted either by phone or in person, preferably during the first week after their quit date. A second follow-up should occur within the first month. During follow-up, a patient's successes are congratulated and reinforced, the use of FDA-approved pharmacologic adjuncts is monitored, and patient concerns and struggles are addressed. Patients should be queried about problems encountered in maintaining abstinence and any future concerns. Four key issues that can arise include weight gain, negative mood or depression, prolonged withdrawal symptoms, and the need for additional support. The dentist and office team may respond with suggestions regarding exercise and diet, alterations to the nicotine replacement dosage, and/or additional phone calls and support. The patient may need a referral to a more intensive program or to a specialist who will prescribe additional medications for mood alteration.

Throughout follow-up, the benefits of cessation must be reinforced and any success (eg, even 1 day without cigarettes) must be congratulated. By asking open-ended questions (eg, "How has stopping smoking helped you?"), the clinician encourages patients to speak openly and freely. This type of dialogue is a key component of relapse prevention. The more patients are able to elicit the benefits of their behavior change, the more they own the process and acknowledge themselves as nonusers.

Most relapse occurs within the first 3 months after quitting; therefore, close monitoring during this time is critical. Patient skill in relapse prevention, although specifically addressed during follow-up, can be developed during the initial appointment. Patients who have had previous quit attempts should be asked, "What happened?" The answer to this type of question can help patients recognize danger situations (eg, emotional upsets, drinking alcohol) and develop coping skills. Patients also need to be informed about the nature of withdrawal and the addictive quality of tobacco.

In the event that a patient does relapse, it should be viewed as a learning experience. The causes of the relapse must be determined, alternative courses discussed, and a recommitment to abstinence established. The dental team's social support, patient skills training, and problem-solving techniques, as well as the use of an FDA-approved pharmacologic agent, are the most effective treatment strategies. When more intensive counseling is warranted and the patient is referred out, the dental practice still should stay abreast of the patient's cessation activities.

As with any protocol, individualization is essential. Special considerations should be followed for adolescents and geriatric and pregnant patients regarding prescribing. The dentist must be aware of any adverse effects, precautions, and contraindications for any pharmacologic adjuncts. Close monitoring of patients ensures sound risk management.

Summary

Since over 50% of tobacco-using patients seek dental care on an annual basis, dentists and the entire oral health team can be instrumental in curbing the incidence of tobacco-induced oral cancer. By instituting the strategies described here and incorporating them into day-to-day practice activities, the team can help many patients in their efforts to abstain from tobacco use. The measures described are brief, effective, and scientifically sound. With the exception of prescription writing, they can be shared by the entire dental team. Oral cancer can be a devastating and disfiguring disease; the efforts of the dentist and the oral health team can help minimize its incidence and effects. A few minutes spent in questioning, advising, assisting, and monitoring tobacco-using patients can promote practice satisfaction and patient well-being.

References

1. Christen AG, McDonald JL, Christen JA. The impact of tobacco use and cessation on nonmalignant and precancerous oral and dental diseases and conditions. Indianapolis: Indiana School of Dentistry, 1991.

2. Mecklenburg RE, Greenspan D, Kleinman DV, et al. Tobacco effects in the mouth. US Dept Health and Human Services, publication 92-3330. Washington DC: Government Printing Office, 1992.

3. National Cancer Institute. Cancer Statistics Review 1973–1987. US Dept Health and Human Services, publication 88-2789. Washington DC: Government Printing Office, 1989.

4. US Department of Health and Human Services. Smokeless tobacco or health. US Dept Health and Human Services, publication 93-3461. Washington DC: Government Printing Office, 1992.

5. Winn DM, Blot WJ, Shy CM, Pickle LC, Toledo A, Fraumen JF Jr. Snuff dipping and oral cancer among women in the southern United States. N Engl J Med 1981;304:745–749.

6. Cancer Facts and Figures 1998. American Cancer Society, Inc. Atlanta, GA.

7. US Department of Health and Human Services. Cigars: Health effects and trends. US Dept Health and Human Services, publication 98-4302. Washington DC: Government Printing Office, 1998.

8. US Centers for Disease Control and Prevention. Cigarette smoking attributable mortality and years of potential life loss - United States, 1990. MMWR 1994; 43 (no. SS1):1–8.

9. Mecklenburg RE, Christen AG, Gerbert B, Gift HC, Glynn TJ, Jones RB, et al. How to help your patients stop using tobacco: National Cancer Institute manual for the oral health team. US Dept Health and Human Services, publication 93-3191. Washington DC: Government Printing Office, 1993.

10. US Department of Health and Human Services. Clinical practices guideline number 18: Smoking cessation. US Dept Health and Human Services, publication 96-0692. Washington DC: Government Printing Office, 1996:19–34.

11. United States Public Health Service. Healthy People 2000: National Health Promotion and Disease Prevention Objectives. US Dept Health and Human Services, publication 91-50212. Washington DC: Government Printing Office, 1990.

12. Tomar SL, Husten CG, Manley MW. Do dentists and physicians advise tobacco users to quit? J Am Dent Assoc 1996;127:259–265.

13. Dolan TA, McGorray SP, Grinstead-Skigen CL, Mecklenburg R. Tobacco control activities in dental practices. J Am Dent Assoc 1997;128:1669–1679.

14. Fried JL, Cohen LA. Maryland dentists' attitudes regarding tobacco issues. Clin Prev Dent 1992;14:10–16.

15. Cohen SJ, Stookey GK, Katz BP, Drook CA, Christen AG. Helping smokers quit: A randomized controlled trial with private practice dentists. J Am Dent Assoc 1989;118:41–45.

16. Martin LM, Bouquot JE, Wingo PA, Health CW. Cancer prevention in the dental practice: Oral cancer screening and tobacco cessation advice. J Public Health Dent 1996;56:336–340.

17. Severson HH, Eakin EG, Steven VJ, Lichtenstein E. Dental office practices for tobacco users: Independent practice and HMO clinics. Am J Public Health 1990;12:1503–1505.

18. Fiore MC. The new vital sign, assessing, and documenting smoking status. JAMA 1991;266:3183–3184.

19. Mecklenburg RE. Tobacco: Addiction, oral health and cessation. Quintessence Int 1998;29:250–252.

20. Kottke TE, Solberg LI, Brekke ML, Conn SA, Maxwell P, Brekke MJ. A controlled trial to integrate smoking cessation advice into primary care practice: Doctors helping smokers, round III. J Fam Pract 1992;34: 701–708.

21. Somerman M, Mecklenburg RE. Cessation of tobacco. In: ADA Guide to Dental Therapeutics. Chicago: American Dental Association, 1998:505–516.

22. Carpenter RD, Yellowitz JA, Goodman HS. Oral cancer mortality in Maryland. MD Med J 1993;42: 1105–1109.

23. Blot WJ, McLaughlin JK, Winn DM, Austin DF, Greenberg RS, Preston-Martin S, et al. Smoking and drinking in relation to oral and pharyngeal cancer. Cancer Res 1988;48:3282–3287.

24. Silverman S, Shillitoe EJ. Etiology and predisposing factors. In: Silverman S (ed). Oral Cancer, ed 3. Atlanta, GA: American Cancer Society, 1989:7–39.

25. Kleinman DV, Crossett LS, Ries LAG, Goldberg HL, Lockwood SA, Swango PA, et al (eds). Cancers of the Oral Cavity and Pharynx: A Statistics Review Monograph 1973–1987. Bethesda, MD: National Cancer Institute, 1991.

26. Silverman S. Epidemiology. In: Silverman S (ed). Oral Cancer, ed 3. Atlanta, GA: American Cancer Society, 1989:1–7.

27. US Centers for Disease Control and Prevention. Preventing Tobacco Use Among Young People: A Report of the Surgeon General. Washington DC: US Depart Health and Human Services, 1994.

28. Gritz ER. Cigarette smoking by adolescent females: Implications for health and behavior. Women Health 1984;9:103–115.

29. Benowitz NL. Pharmacologic aspects of cigarette smoking and nicotine addiction. N Engl J Med 1988;319:1318–1330.

30. Sorensen G, Pechacek T. Attitudes toward smoking cessation among men and women. J Behav Med 1987;10:129–137.

31. Leischow SJ, Stitzer ML. Smoking cessation and weight gain. Br J Addict 1991;86:577–581.

32. Hatsukami D, Skoog K, Allen S, Bliss R. Gender and the effects of different doses of nicotine gum on tobacco withdrawal symptoms. Exp Clin Psychopharmacol 1995;3:163–173..

33. Hurt RD, Sachs DP, Glover ED, Offard KP, Johnston JA. A comparison of sustained-release buproprion and placebo for smoking cessation. N Engl J Med 1997;337:1195–1202.

CHAPTER 19

Chemoprevention

Barbara A. Conley, MD

Carcinogenesis is postulated to be a multi-step process. Initiation events, which result in DNA damage, are followed by a reversible promotion phase, and finally by progression to full malignant cancer.[1] These stages can sometimes be observed histologically. Premalignant intraepithelial neoplasia (dysplasia), a localized abnormal proliferation of cells that precedes malignant invasion, may represent a stage of carcinogenesis that is reversible.[2]

head and neck, a few agents do hold some promise. These include retinoids, nonsteroidal anti-inflammatory agents (cyclooxygenase inhibitors), vitamin E, interferons, and green tea components. This chapter reviews the current status of clinical trials for prevention of the initial head and neck tumor in patients at high risk for developing the disease, as well as trials for prevention of second primary tumors after an initial tumor has received curative treatment.

Definition

Chemoprevention refers to the administration of an agent to prevent a cancer from occurring. The agent can be a drug or a natural product. Candidate agents for chemoprevention should have certain characteristics. The agent must be easy to administer, cause little or no toxicity, cause no long-term adverse sequelae, be affordable, and, ideally, need to be administered only for a short time, relative to a lifetime. Few agents have met these criteria. However, for prevention of cancers of the

Chemoprevention Research

One of the major targets for chemopreventive research is cancer of the upper aerodigestive tract. Patients who have been diagnosed with a single squamous cell carcinoma in the head and neck region have a 4% to 6% chance per year of developing a second tumor in the upper aerodigestive tract, including the oral, oropharyngeal, laryngeal, lung, and esophageal areas.[1] This behavior is an example of the field cancerization theory, as defined by Slaughter et al.[3] In addition, the head and neck area may manifest premalignant changes, such as leukoplakia or erythroplakia, which increase the risk of developing a cancer. Patients with dysplasia, for example, may have up to a 36% chance of eventually developing a cancer in the head and neck region.[4] While oral leukoplakia without dysplasia is considered a premalignant lesion, the rate of transformation to malignancy is generally lower than that for dysplastic lesions and ranges from 1.4% to 4.6% in published series.[5,6]

Leukoplakia

The treatment of a patient with leukoplakia can be difficult. Erythroplakia has a rate of malignant transformation and a rate of associated carcinoma (in situ or invasive) high enough to make surgical removal standard. However, surgical removal may not even be possible in patients with extensive or panleukoplakia. Even when removed, the lesions may recur. Moreover, patients may have malignant change in an area without leukoplakia, making it difficult to know where to biopsy to detect an early cancer. Patients with leukoplakia and/or dysplasia are therefore good candidates for clinical trials of putative chemoprevention agents.

Several trials of retinoid use in oral leukoplakia have been performed:

- Stich et al[7] compared 6 months of treatment with vitamin A versus placebo in Indian betel nut chewers. This trial found regression of leukoplakia associated with vitamin A treatment, as well as a reduction in the formation of new leukoplakias when compared to patients who were randomized to placebo. This effect occurred despite the continuation of betel nut chewing by the patients.

- Hong et al[8] randomly assigned patients with leukoplakia to treatment with isotretinoin (an isomer of all-*trans*-retinoic acid) 1 to 2 mg/kg per day for 3 months, or to placebo. Twenty-three of the 44 patients had dysplasia. Dysplasia was reversed in 54% of the patients who were randomized to isotretinoin versus 10% of those randomized to placebo. However, responses were temporary and relapse occurred once the treatment stopped. Toxicity (mucocutaneous dryness and hypertriglyceridemia) prompted dose reduction in nearly half of the patients.
- In a follow-up study,[9] 70 patients with leukoplakia were treated for 3 months with isotretinoin. If there was no progression (59 patients), patients were randomized to treatment with either beta carotene or low-dose isotretinoin for 9 months. The rate of progression in the patients randomized to isotretinoin was lower than that for those randomized to beta carotene (8% versus 55%, $P < 0.001$).
- Koch[10] treated patients with leukoplakia with either all-*trans*-retinoic acid, isotretinoin, or an aromatic retinoid. Early responses occurred in 59% to 91% of patients and were durable for up to 6 years with continued treatment. However, relapse occurred when treatment stopped.
- Garewal et al[11] treated patients with beta carotene and observed responses in 9 of 11 patients with dysplasia. However, 8 of the 11 relapsed after treatment stopped.
- Stich et al[12] compared 6 months of treatment with beta carotene, beta carotene with vitamin A, and placebo in Indian betel nut chewers who had elevated frequencies of micronucleated cells, which is an indicator of DNA damage. Both treatment arms produced more remissions (14% to 28%) than the placebo arm, as well as reductions in the frequency of micronuclei, without toxicity.

- Chiesa et al[13] randomized patients with leukoplakia to treatment with fenretinide (a semisynthetic retinoid) or to placebo after complete surgical excision of the leukoplakia. Fewer recurrences were observed in the fenretinide-treated group, and toxicity was mild. In eight patients with either nonoperable lichen planus or leukoplakia treated with topical fenretinide, all had significant reduction in the size of the lesion.

Currently, the National Cancer Institute Division of Cancer Prevention is sponsoring a randomized trial of fenretinide versus placebo in patients with oral dysplasia. To date, however, no trial has demonstrated a permanent effect of the chemopreventive. Rather, the agent must be given continuously to maintain the effect.

Prevention of second primary carcinoma

The second population that is appropriate for chemoprevention clinical trials are those patients who have had definitive treatment for an early squamous cell carcinoma of the head and neck or lung. Early lesions are likely to be cured by definitive surgery or radiation therapy, and therefore the patient has many years of risk in which to develop a second primary tumor of the upper aerodigestive tract.

To date, only isotretinoin has shown significant activity in prevention of second primary tumors in patients who have had an initial squamous cell carcinoma of the head and neck. Hong et al[14] and Benner et al[15] reported a trial of isotretinoin, 1 to 2 mg/kg, versus placebo in 103 patients who were curatively treated for squamous cell carcinoma of the head and neck. About half of the patients had at least stage III cancers initially. There was a

statistically significant reduction in the rate of second primary cancers in the group treated with isotretinoin versus those treated with placebo (14% versus 31%, respectively) with a nearly 5-year median follow-up time. However, there was no difference in overall survival between the two groups. Additionally, treatment with isotretinoin did not affect the likelihood of recurrence of the original tumor. The effect was seen during treatment only, with rates of developing second primary tumors in patients treated with isotretinoin approaching those of the placebo group once treatment stopped. These results were promising, even though a significant number of patients needed dose reductions for toxicity, and approximately one third of the patients did not complete the prescribed 1-year treatment course.

This population remains a priority for the development of effective agents that reduce the morbidity and mortality from aerodigestive tract cancer. Currently, a national trial in the United States randomizes patients with curatively treated stage I or II squamous cell carcinoma of the head and neck to either isotretinoin or to placebo. The accrual to this trial will be completed in 1999, but the analysis will not be complete for several years thereafter.

A French trial randomized patients with early oropharyngeal or oral cancer to either etretinate (a retinoid) or to placebo. However, this trial did not find a difference in the rate of second primary tumors in this population.[16] A large randomized trial of vitamin A in the form of retinyl-palmitate, N-acetylcysteine, or the combination of the two drugs versus placebo (EUROSCAN) has completed accrual in Europe. This trial accepted about 2,000 patients with curatively treated oral, laryngeal, or lung cancer. Analysis of the trial is not yet complete.

Promising Agents for Chemoprevention of Head and Neck Cancer

Retinoids

Several retinoids have been studied for prevention of head and neck cancer as well as for other cancers. Retinoids are necessary for normal fetal development, as well as for normal reproductive function and for vision. The mechanism of action of these compounds for chemoprevention is not well understood. Studies have documented lower beta carotene (a precursor of vitamin A) serum concentrations in patients who develop cancer of the head and neck, than in patients who do not develop these cancerous tumors.[17] Retinoids can act through induction of differentiation and can inhibit proliferation, as well as cause programmed cell death.[18] Cellular binding proteins exist for retinoids, although their function has not been elucidated. Nuclear retinoic acid receptors bind to certain areas of DNA and presumably interact with the genome to express or repress certain genes important for the development of malignancy.[18] The function of these genes has not yet been made clear. However, down-regulation of the retinoic acid receptor beta has been correlated with malignant progression, and it can be restored by treatment with retinoids.[19] Various isomers of retinoic acid have been studied for activity in cancer treatment and/or prevention. These include all-*trans*-retinoic acid, 9-*cis*-retinoic acid, and 13-*cis*-retinoic acid (isotretinoin). In addition, retinoids that do not seem to bind with great affinity to the nuclear retinoic acid receptor (fenretinide), as well as those that are selective for certain receptors, may show promise in this area. Vitamin A, or retinol, is toxic to the liver, and therefore is not used in these trials. Vitamin A is a precursor of all-*trans*-retinoic acid, 9-*cis*-retinoic acid, and 13-*cis*-retinoic acid.

Beta carotene

Beta carotene is one of several carotenoids in the body and is a precursor of vitamin A. It is found in leafy green vegetables and yellow and orange fruits and vegetables, and it is also available in tablet form. To some extent it is converted to vitamin A in the body and is not associated with hypervitaminosis A syndrome. Several studies have noted lower blood levels of beta carotene in patients who develop aerodigestive tract cancers compared to patients who do not develop cancer.[17] These findings led to a hypothesis that a beta carotene deficiency may predispose cancer formation. Although there is little toxicity associated with beta carotene administration, its use as a chemopreventive agent is experimental and has been associated with regression of leukoplakia, but also with increased cancer incidence. The mechanism of action of beta carotene as a chemopreventive agent may involve antioxidant mechanisms as well as inhibition of free radical reactions.[20]

N-Acetylcysteine

N-Acetylcysteine is an antioxidant and free-radical scavenger that has shown chemopreventive activity in lung and tracheal tumors in animals.[21] These data, as well as its activity as a detoxifying agent and its lack of major toxicity, have made this agent a candidate for chemoprevention trials.

Nonsteroidal anti-inflammatory agents

In animal studies, nonsteroidal anti-inflammatory agents (NSAIDs) have chemopreventive activity in several tissues and have shown activity in tumor inhibition in preclinical head and neck cancer models.[22] Because these compounds may be inhibitors of proliferation, they may be useful as chemopreventive agents. However, many members of this class of agents have the side effect of unpredictable massive gastrointestinal bleeding in a minority of patients. Selective inhibitors of cyclooxygenase 2 (COX-2), an inducible enzyme, are being investigated for antitumor activity and lack of gastrointestinal toxicity.

Vitamin E

Vitamin E has been effective in reducing oral cancer progression in a hamster buccal pouch model.[23] Epidemiologic studies have noted an inverse relationship between serum vitamin E levels and the development of oral and oropharyngeal cancer.[17] In addition, oral vitamin E has been shown to reduce oral mucosal micronuclei frequency, although no clinical effect was demonstrated.[24] Its mechanism of action is postulated to be as an antioxidant agent. It can ameliorate some of the toxicities of all-*trans*-retinoic acid. Combinations of vitamin E and retinoids are currently being studied in chemoprevention clinical trials.

Interferons

Interferons have shown additive or synergistic antitumor effects in combination with retinoids.[25] However, administration of interferons, to date, requires frequent subcutaneous injections and is accompanied by a mild to moderate flulike syndrome. These characteristics make interferons undesirable chemopreventive agents.

Curcumin

Curcumin is the major component of turmeric, which is widely used in curry. Curcumin has inhibited carcinogen-induced tumorigenesis in an oral cancer model[26] and is nontoxic. This agent is under consideration as a cancer preventive.

Green tea

Green tea is consumed worldwide and is especially popular in the Far East. Epidemiologic studies have found that consumption of green tea is associated with a lower incidence of cancers such as gastric and esophageal cancer.[27] Epigallocatechin-3-gallate (EGCG) is the major constituent of green tea, and this compound has been shown to be growth inhibitory in an in vitro model of oral carcinogenesis,[27] at concentrations that could be achieved by oral ingestion of green tea. This compound is being evaluated for clinical chemoprevention trials.

Other Chemoprevention Trials

Breast cancer

Two recent clinical trials deserve mention. The Breast Cancer Prevention Trial performed by the National Surgical Adjuvant Breast and Bowel Program in the United States compared tamoxifen (an antiestrogen compound) versus placebo in 13,388 women at high risk for invasive breast cancer. This trial was recently terminated early, after demonstration of a 49% reduction in the risk of breast cancer development in the experimental group.[28] Another trial, evaluating raloxifene (a selective estrogen receptor molecule, or SERM) versus placebo for prevention of osteoporotic fractures also found that breast cancers were less frequent in the women who received raloxifene.[29] A trial comparing tamoxifen and raloxifene for the prevention of breast cancer in women at high risk of this disease will begin shortly.

Lung cancer

Unfortunately, two large chemoprevention trials for lung cancer point out the pitfalls in chemoprevention research. Plasma retinol had been shown to be lower in patients with lung cancer than in those who did not have cancer. However, a trial from Finland, the Alpha-Tocopherol-Beta Carotene (ATBC) Trial, randomized male smokers between the ages of 50 and 69 to alpha tocopherol (50 mg daily), beta carotene (20 mg daily), the two combined, or neither agent. After entry of 29,133 patients, those who had been randomized to beta carotene had an increased risk of lung cancer and of death.[30] This was a puzzling result, but it was confirmed when a large US trial, the Beta-Carotene and Retinol Efficacy Trial (CARET), closed after interim analysis indicated a similar result. This trial randomized 18,314 men and women at high risk of developing lung cancer to 30 mg beta carotene plus 25,000 IU retinyl-palmitate daily or to placebo. The trial was stopped 21 months early because of clear evidence there was no benefit to the chemoprevention regimen. In fact, patients who were randomized to the chemoprevention agents had 28% more lung cancers and 17% more deaths than the placebo group.[31] Based on the results of these two trials, it was concluded that patients who are at high

risk of lung cancer, ie, current smokers and asbestos-exposed workers, should be discouraged from taking beta carotene and/or vitamin A supplements.

Summary

Chemoprevention research represents a promising early intervention in the cancer pathway. Development of such agents has been difficult due to lack of preclinical models and lack of specificity from epidemiologic studies. At present, chemoprevention treatments remain experimental. Chemopreventive agents should only be given in well-controlled clinical trials in which patients can be observed closely for adverse reactions or the development of cancer.

References

1. Lippman SM, Benner SE, Hong WK. Cancer chemoprevention. J Clin Oncol 1994;12:851.

2. Boone CW, Kelloff GJ, Steele VE. Natural history of intraepithelial neoplasia in humans with implications for cancer chemopreventive strategy. Cancer Res 1992;52:1651.

3. Slaughter DL, Southwick HW, Smejkal W. Field cancerization in oral stratified squamous epithelium: Clinical implications of multicentric origin. Cancer 1953;6:963.

4. Lumerman H, Freedman P, Kerpel S. Oral epithelial dysplasia and the development of invasive squamous cell carcinoma. Oral Surg Oral Med Oral Pathol 1995;79:321.

5. Pindborg JJ, Jolst O, Renstrup G, Roed-Petersen B. Studies with oral leukoplakia: A preliminary report on the period prevalence of malignant transformation in leukoplakia based on a followup study of 248 patients. J Am Dent Assoc 1968;78:767–771.

6. Banoczy J. Oral Leukoplakia. Boston: Martinus Nijhoff, 1982:15–27.

7. Stich HF, Hornby AP, Mathew B, Sankaranarayanan R, Nair MK. Response of oral leukoplakia to the administration of vitamin A. Cancer Lett 1988;40:93–101.

8. Hong WK, Endicott J, Itri LM, Doos W, Batsakis JG, Bell R, et al. 13-cis retinoic acid in the treatment of oral leukoplakia. N Engl J Med 1986;315:1501–1505.

9. Lippman SM, Batsakis JG, Toth BB, Weber RS, Lee JJ, Martin JW, et al. Comparison of low-dose isotretinoin with beta carotene to prevent oral carcinogenesis. N Engl J Med 1993;328:15–20.

10. Koch HF. Biochemical treatment of precancerous oral lesions: The effectiveness of various analogues of retinoic acid. J Maxillofac Surg 1978;6:59.

11. Garewal HS, Meyskens FL Jr, Killen D, Reeves D, Kiersch TA, Elletson H, et al. Response of oral leukoplakia to beta-carotene. J Clin Oncol 1990;8:1715–1720.

12. Stich HF, Rosin MP, Hornby P, Mathew B, Sankaranarayanan R, Nair MK. Remission of oral leukoplakias and micronuclei in tobacco/betel quid chewers treated with beta-carotene and with beta-carotene plus vitamin A. Eur J Cancer 1988;42:195.

13. Chiesa F, Tradati N, Marazza M, Rossi N, Boracchi P, Mariani L, et al. Prevention of local relapse and new localisations of oral leukoplakias with the synthetic retinoid fenretinide (4-HPR). Preliminary results. Eur J Cancer B Oral Oncol 1992;28B:97–102.

14. Hong WK, Lippman SM, Itri LM, Karp DD, Lee JS, Byers RM, et al. Prevention of second primary tumors with isotretinoin in squamous cell carcinoma of the head and neck. N Engl J Med 1990;323:795–801.

15. Benner SE, Pajak TF, Lippman SM, Earley C, Hong WK. Prevention of second primary tumors with isotretinoin in patients with squamous cell carcinoma of the head and neck: Long-term follow-up. J Natl Cancer Inst 1994;86:140–141.

16. Bolla M, Lefur R, Ton Van J, Domenge C, Badet JM, Koskas Y, et al. Prevention of second primary tumours with etretinate in squamous cell carcinoma of the oral cavity and oropharynx. Results of a multicentric double-blind randomized study. Eur J Cancer 1994;30A: 727–729.

17. Zheng W, Blot WJ, Diamond EL, Norkus EP, Spate V, Morris JS, et al. Serum micronutrients and the subsequent risk of oral and pharyngeal cancer. Cancer Res 1993;53:795–798.

18. Smith MA, Parkinson DR, Cheson BD, Friedman MA. Retinoids in cancer therapy. J Clin Oncol 1992;10:839.

19. Lotan R, Xu XC, Lippman SM, Ro JY, Lee JS, Lee JJ, et al. Suppression of retinoic acid receptor beta in premalignant oral lesions and its upregulation by isotretinoin. N Engl J Med 1995;332:1405–1410.

20. Sies H, Stahl W, Sundquist AR. Antioxidant functions of vitamins: Vitamins E and C, beta carotene and other carotenoids. Ann N Y Acad Sci 1992;669:7.

21. deVries N, Pastorino U, van Zandwijk N. Chemoprevention of second primary tumours in head and neck cancer in Europe: EUROSCAN. Eur J Cancer B Oral Oncol 1994;30B:367.

22. Kelloff GJ, Boone CW, Crowell JA, Steele VE, Lubet R, Sigman CC. Chemopreventive drug development: Perspectives and progress. Cancer Epidemiol Biomarkers Prev 1994;3:85.

23. Papadimitrakopoulou VA, Shin D, Hong WK. Chemoprevention of head and neck cancer. In: Harrison LB, Sessions RB, Hong WK (eds). Head and Neck Cancer, a Multidisciplinary Approach. Philadelphia: Lippincott-Raven, 1999:49–75.

24. Benner SE, Wargovich MJ, Lippman SM, Fisher R, Velasco M, Winn RJ, et al. Reduction in oral mucosa micronuclei frequency following alpha-tocopherol treatment of oral leukoplakia. Cancer Epidemiol Biomarkers Prev 1994;3:73–76.

25. Lippman SM, Parkinson DR, Itri LM, Weber RS, Shantz SP, Ota DM, et al. 13-cis retinoic acid plus interferon-alpha-2a: Effective combination therapy for advanced squamous cell carcinoma of the skin. J Natl Cancer Inst 1992;84:241–245.

26. Tanaka T, Makita H, Ohnishi M, Hirose Y, Wang A, Mori H, et al. Chemoprevention of 4-nitroquinoline1-oxide-induced oral carcinogenesis by dietary curcumin and hesperidin: Comparison with the protective effect of beta-carotene. Cancer Res 1994;54: 4653–4659.

27. Khafif A, Schantz SP, Al-Rawi M, Edelstein D, Sacks PG. Green tea regulates cell cycle progression in oral leukoplakia. Head Neck 1998;20:528.

28. Fisher B, Costantino JP, Wickerham DL, Redmond CK, Kavanah M, Cronin WM, et al. Tamoxifen for prevention of breast cancer: Report of the National Surgical Adjuvant Breast and Bowel Project P-1 study. J Natl Cancer Inst 1998;90:1371–1388.

29. Cummings SR, Norton L, Eckert S, Grady D, Cauley J, Knickerbocker R, et al. Raloxifene reduces the risk of breast cancer and may decrease the risk of endometrial cancer in postmenopausal women. Two-year findings from the Multiple Outcomes of Raloxifene Evaluation (MORE) trial. Proc Am Soc Clin Oncol 1998;17:2a.

30. The Alpha-Tocopherol, Beta Carotene Cancer Prevention Study Group. The effect of vitamin E and beta carotene on the incidence of lung cancer and other cancers in male smokers. N Engl J Med 1994;330:1029.

31. Omenn GS, Goodman GE, Thornquist MD, Balmes J, Cullen MR, Glass A, et al. Risk factors for lung cancer and for intervention effects in CARET, the Beta-Carotene and Retinol Efficacy Trial. J Natl Cancer Inst 1996;88:1550–1559.

Index

Spindle cell carcinoma, 66–67
Split-thickness skin grafting, for reconstruction of oral lining tissues, 107
Squamous cell carcinoma
  allelic losses associated with, 12–13
  basaloid, 67, 67f
  biopsy for, 43
  cortactin in, 15
  description of, 4
  early detection of, 21
  human papillomavirus and, 4, 10
  illustration of, 52f
  oral lichen planus and, 57, 58f
  risk factors
    alcohol consumption, 7, 9–10, 22
    cigarette smoking, 6, 22
  of tongue, 104f
  unresectable, 128
Stomatitis, 135–136, 136f. See also
    Mucositis.
Submandibular glands
  examination procedure for, 33f
  lymphatic system of, 28t
  radiation therapy effects, 119–120, 153
Submental gland
  examination procedure for, 33f
  lymphatic system of, 28t
Subperiosteal bone, in Ewing's sarcoma, 39
Sucralfate, 142, 152
Suicidal ideation, 205, 207, 212
Superficial cervical lymph nodes, examination procedure for, 30f
Supraclavicular area, examination procedure for, 30f
Supraomohyoid neck dissection, 90, 91f
Surgical guide, for implant-supported prostheses, 185, 192, 193f
Surgical management. See also specific
    surgical procedure.
  access, 83f–86f, 83–84
  conservative ablation
    marginal resection technique, 87, 88f
    for neck, 87, 90–91
  margins, 84, 87
  overview of, 81–82
  for recurrent disease, 90–91
  TMN staging system, 81, 82t
Surgical reconstruction. See
    Reconstructive surgery.
Surveillance, Epidemiology and End
    Results program, 4
Survival rates, 81
Swallowing. See also Dysphagia.
  illustration of, 199f
  phases of, 197

physiology of, 197
rehabilitation of
  pretreatment evaluation, 201–202
  speech language pathologist's
    involvement in, 198, 200–201
  strategies, 199b, 201
  surgical impact on, 200b

T

Taste buds, radiation therapy effects on, 119
Teeth, radiologic studies of, 39, 40f
Temporalis muscle flap, for reconstruction of oral lining tissues, 107
Temporomandibular joint, examination procedure for, 31f
Thyroid gland, examination procedure for, 31f
TMN staging system, 81, 82t
Tobacco use. See also Cigarette smoking.
  assessment form for, 225f
  cessation of
    Agency for Health Care Policy and
      Research guidelines, 222t–223t
    clinic/practice environment for, 221, 224
    dentist's role in, 219–221
    pharmacologic methods, 227t
    step-based strategy for, 224, 226–229
    studies regarding, 219–220
  smokeless
    commercial forms, 57
    lesions associated with, 57, 59, 59f
    leukoplakia risks associated with, 59
    placement variations, 59
Toluidine blue stain, 44f–45f, 44–45
Tongue
  cancer incidence of, 197
  examination procedure for, 34f
  leukoplakia of, 49, 50f, 52f
  lichen planus of, 58f
  muscular function of, 101
  necrosis of, 151f
  radiation therapy principles, 116
  resection of, 200–201
  in speech production, 197
  surgical access, 83
  verruca vulgaris of, 62f
Tonsils, examination procedure for, 34f
Topical anesthetics, for mucositis, 142
Transoral alveolar sequestrectomy, 172
Trismus, 153, 161
Tumoritis, 118

Two-punch theory, for tongue reconstruction, 101

U

Ultrasound, 42
University of Maryland studies, 7–8

V

Vascularized bone transfer, for
    mandibular reconstruction, 97
Venereal warts. See Condyloma acuminatum.
Verruca vulgaris, 61, 62f
Verrucous carcinoma
  anatomic sites, 65
  characteristics of, 65
  description of, 10
  histologic findings, 65
  illustration of, 60f
  lesions, 65, 66f
  metastasis, 65
  smokeless tobacco lesions and, 59
  treatment of, 65–66
Verrucous leukoplakia, proliferative
  characteristics of, 61
  illustration of, 60f
Vitamin A, for leukoplakia, 232
Vitamin E, chemopreventive uses of, 235
Vocal tract, 197, 198f

W

Women, 5t, 9

X

Xerostomia
  in chemotherapy patients, 138–139
  clinical manifestations, 153–154
  from radiation therapy
    description of, 119–120
    prilocaine for, 120
  in radiation therapy patients, 153–155
  treatment of, 145, 154–155

Z

Zilactin, 142
Zyban. See Bupropion hydrochloride.